PocketRadiologist®
Obstetrics
Top 100 Diagnoses

Specialties included in the PocketRadiologist® series

Abdominal, Top 100 Diagnoses

Brain, Top 100 Diagnoses

Cardiac, Top 100 Diagnoses

Chest, Top 100 Diagnoses

Head & Neck, Top 100 Diagnoses

Musculoskeletal, Top 100 Diagnoses

Pediatrics, Top 100 Diagnoses

PedsNeuro, Top 100 Diagnoses

Spine, Top 100 Diagnoses

Temporal Bone, Top 100 Diagnoses

Vascular, Top 100 Diagnoses

and

Interventional, Top 100 Procedures

Holoprosencephaly

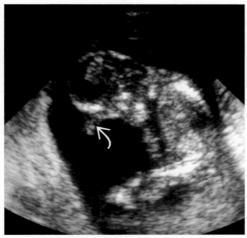

Alobar holoprosencephaly. A midline sagittal view in the same fetus shows a fleshy proboscis projecting from the mid-face (arrow).

o Mild forms often difficult to detect

Ultrasound Findings

• Vary according to severity of malformation
• Fused thalami
• **Absent cavum septi pellucidi** in all forms
• Falx absent/incomplete
• Absent 3rd ventricle
• **Dorsal sac**
  o Herniation of telea choroidea
  o Cystic extension of monoventricle
    ▪ Can be large
• Absent corpus callosum
• Facial defects
  o **Cebocephaly**
    ▪ Cyclopia
    ▪ Hypotelorism
    ▪ Proboscis located above eyes with absent nose
    ▪ Single nostril
    ▪ Flattened nose
  o **Midline** facial cleft

MR Findings

• Very helpful when US is equivocal
• Fused thalami and fornices more easily demonstrated

Imaging Recommendations

• Look for associated chromosomal abnormalities and syndromes
• MRI for difficult cases

Differential Diagnosis

Hydranancephaly

• No cerebral tissue
• **Falx present**

Holoprosencephaly

- **Normal facial development**
Aqueductal Stenosis
- Cavum septi pellucidi present
- Dilated 3rd ventricle
- Thalami not fused
Arachnoid Cyst
- Can be confused with dorsal sac
- Ventricular system may be dilated but otherwise normal
Porencephaly
- Usually asymmetric ventricular enlargement
- May see evidence of residual hematoma which evolves over time
Agenesis of the Corpus Callosum
- May mimic lobar holoprosencephaly
- 3rd ventricle present but abnormally high
- Ventricles parallel and teardrop-shaped (colpocephaly)
- MRI may be needed to differentiate

Pathology
General
- Associated with multiple syndromes including
  o Smith-Lemli-Opitz syndrome
  o Aicardi syndrome
  o Fryn syndrome
- Genetics
  o Most are sporadic
  o Autosomal recessive, dominant, and X-linked forms described
  o 11 different chromosomes implicated
  o Seen in T13, T18, triploidy
- Embryology
  o Failure of normal cleavage of prosencephalon (4-6 weeks)
- Epidemiology
  o 1:16,000 births
  o More common in utero (1:250 in terminated pregnancies)

Clinical Issues
Presentation
- May have an abnormal triple screen (T13)
- May be diagnosed in 1st trimester
Treatment
- Karyotype
- Termination offered
- Fetal intervention not indicated
Prognosis
- Dependent on type and severity
- Alobar usually fatal in neonatal period
- Other forms varying degrees of mental retardation and developmental delay

Selected References
1. McGahan JP et al: Sonography of facial features of alobar and semilobar holoprosencephaly. AJR Am J Roentgenol 154:143-8, 1990
2. McGahan JP et al: Congenital cerebrospinal fluid-containing intracranial abnormalities: A sonographic classification. J Clin Ultrasound 16:531-44, 1988
3. Pilu G et al: Criteria for the prenatal diagnosis of holoprosencephaly. Am J Perinatol 4:41-9, 1987

Hydranencephaly

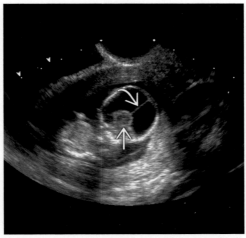

Hydranencephaly. Endovaginal ultrasound of 14 week fetus shows falx (curved arrow) with no cerebral hemisphere tissue. The brain stem (arrow) bulges into the fluid-filled supratentorial space mimicking fused thalami in holoprosencephaly.

Key Facts
- Definition: **Complete destruction of cerebral hemispheres** with normal cerebellum and brainstem
- Classic imaging appearance: Supratentorial space entirely fluid filled
- Confused with hydrocephalus
  - Thin rim of cerebral tissue
- Confused with holoprosencephaly
  - Absent or incomplete falx
  - Often other anomalies
- Evolving hydranencephaly may mimic tumor

Imaging Findings
Ultrasound Findings
- Structural survey normal apart from brain
- Intracranial findings evolve with stage
  - Echogenic mass: Focal hemorrhage
  - Diffuse parenchymal destruction
    - Loss of normal landmarks
    - Diffusely abnormal intracranial echoes
  - Replacement of cerebral hemispheres by fluid
    - End stage of process
    - May be seen at **presentation**
- Best imaging clue
  - Fluid-filled supratentorial space
  - Falx present
  - Normal posterior fossa
MR Findings
- SSFSE
  - Confirms absence of cerebral hemispheres

Hydranencephaly

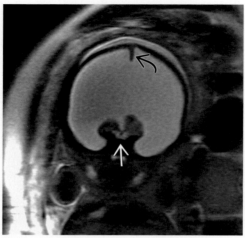

Hydranencephaly. Coronal SSFSE image at 32 weeks gestation shows the brainstem (arrow) bulging into the fluid-filled supratentorial space. No cerebral tissue is identified. Note the presence of a falx (curved arrow). The bulging brainstem can be mistaken for thalamic fusion on ultrasound.

- o Medial temporal lobes may be present
  - ▪ Supplied by posterior circulation
- o If anterior temporal tissue present then severe hydrocephalus
  - ▪ Cortical mantle thinned but present

Imaging Recommendations
- Complete anatomic survey
- **MCA flow** present in hydrocephalus/**absent in hydranencephaly**
- Aim to prove presence/absence cerebral mantle
- MRI to differentiate from severe hydrocephalus

Differential Diagnosis

Hydrocephalus
- Cortical mantle present
- Posterior fossa often abnormal
  - o Dandy-Walker malformation: Posterior fossa cyst
  - o Arnold-Chiari malformation: Obliteration of cisterna magna
- Frequently associated with other structural anomalies
  - o Myelomeningocele
  - o Clubfeet

Holoprosencephaly
- Monoventricle
- Fused thalami
- Frequently associated with abnormal face
  - o Midline facial cleft
  - o Cyclopia
  - o Proboscis
  - o Cebocephaly

Hydranencephaly

Pathology
General
- Fowler type: Proliferative vasculopathy and hydranencephaly-hydrocephaly (PVHH)
  - Characteristic proliferative "glomeruloid" vasculopathy
  - Impairs vascular invasion of cerebral mantle in first trimester
  - Possible mitochondrial dysfunction
- Genetics
  - Consanguineous family with autosomal recessive inheritance
    - Defect mapped to chromosome 16p13.3-12.1
  - Fowler type: Autosomal recessive
- Etiology-Pathogenesis: Proposed etiologies
  - Vascular malformation
    - Carotid webbing
    - Absent internal carotid system
  - Bilateral carotid occlusion
  - Profound fetal hypotension/hypoxia
  - Intrauterine infection
  - Irradiation
  - Coagulation disorders $\Rightarrow$ ICH $\Rightarrow$ cerebral destruction
  - Aggressive tumor may destroy brain $\Rightarrow$ hydranencephaly
- Epidemiology
  - 1:4-10,000 live births
  - 0.6% CNS malformations in perinatal/neonatal autopsy series
  - Scattered case reports of hemi-hydranencephaly
  - Smoking, decreased maternal age increase risk

Clinical Issues
Presentation
- Described as early as 12 weeks
Treatment
- Infection screen
- Coagulation screen
- Consider karyotype
- Offer termination
- If pregnancy progresses: Non-intervention in labor
- Offer cephalocentesis if macrocephaly would preclude vaginal delivery
Prognosis
- Extremely poor
  - 50% live-born infants die in first month
  - 85% mortality by end first year
  - Occasional long term survivors
    - No cognitive function, require institutional care
- Hemihydranencephaly
  - Better prognosis: 4 of 6 reported cases show "mild" developmental delay

Selected References
1. Laurichesse-Delmas H et al: First trimester features of Fowler syndrome (hydrocephaly-hydranencephaly proliferative vasculopathy). Ultrasound Obstet Gynecol 20:612-15, 2002
2. Greco F et al: Hemihydranencephaly: Case report and literature review. J Child Neurol 16:218-21, 2001
3. Kavaslar GN et al: The novel genetic disorder microhydranencephaly maps to chromosome 16p13.3-12.1. Am J Hum Genet 66:1705-9, 2000

Porencephaly

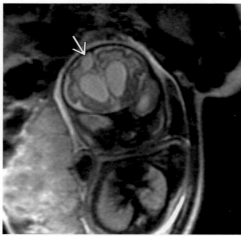

Porencephaly. Coronal SSFSE image from fetal MRI in the third trimester shows hydrocephalus and a porencephalic cyst (arrow) secondary to a thrombosed dural arteriovenous fistula (AVF). AVF is posterior and not visible in this image.

Key Facts
- Definition: Destructive defect in brain parenchyma, may communicate with CSF spaces
- Classic imaging appearance: Cystic brain lesion associated with hydrocephalus but no mass effect
- **Normal development with later destruction**
  - Periventricular leukomalacia
  - Porencephaly
  - Hydranencephaly
- Abnormal development: Not part of porencephaly/hydranencephaly spectrum
  - Neuronal migration disorders
  - Schizencephaly

Imaging Findings
General Features
- Best imaging clue: Intraaxial avascular fluid attenuation structure without mass effect
Ultrasound Findings
- Round or irregular shape
- **No mass effect**
- Hydrocephalus: Parenchymal destruction
- No flow on Doppler
MR Findings
- FMPSPGR
  - High signal blood products ⇒ adjacent hemorrhage
- SSFSE
  - CSF signal in cyst
  - Abnormally high signal adjacent brain parenchyma ⇒ destruction
  - Space not lined with gray matter

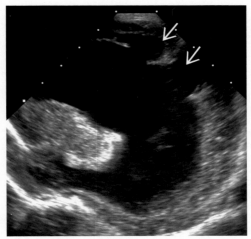

Porencephaly. Neonatal head ultrasound performed on first day of life via anterior fontanelle. Sagittal image of the right lateral ventricle shows hydrocephalus communicating with porencephalic cysts (arrows).

- o Communication with ventricles
- o Low signal blood products

Imaging Recommendations
- Careful survey for other defects
  - o Vascular compromise
    - Renal
    - Extremity
  - o Infection
    - Liver calcifications
    - Intracranial calcifications
    - Hydrops
- Check for placental abruption
- Lesion develops over time
  - o Normal scan at time of "event" **does not** exclude diagnosis
  - o Re-image at 10 to 14 days

Differential Diagnosis

Arachnoid Cyst
- Extraaxial
- Displaces normal brain
- Not associated with destructive process

Schizencephaly
- Cortical cleft lined with gray matter
- Wedge shape rather than round or irregular

Vascular Malformation
- Flow on Doppler
- Vein of Galen aneurysm
  - o Quadrigeminal plate cistern, postero-superior to thalami
- Vascular "steal"/venous hypertension $\Rightarrow$ parenchymal destruction and focal porencephaly **in addition to** AVF

Porencephaly

- Dural Arteriovenous Fistula (AVF)
  - o Extraaxial
  - o Enlarged feeding and draining vessels

Pathology
General
- Genetics
  - o Familial types occur
- Etiology-Pathogenesis
  - o Infection
    - Cytomegalovirus
    - Toxoplasmosis
    - Varicella/Zoster
  - o Vascular: Hypoperfusion
    - Monochorionic twin demise
    - Intracranial hemorrhage
    - Maternal drug use: Cocaine
    - Fetal intervention: Intrauterine transfusion, twin vessel laser coagulation
  - o Syndromic
    - Encephalocraniocutaneous lipomatosis
- Epidemiology
  - o Rare

Clinical Issues
Treatment
- Infection screen
- Evaluate for bleeding diathesis
- Offer termination
  - o Encourage autopsy for definitive diagnosis
- Not indication for early delivery
Prognosis
- Neurodevelopmental outcome poor
- Depends on size and location of cyst
  - o Visual loss
  - o Speech impairment
  - o Hydrocephalus
  - o Sensory/motor deficit
  - o Seizure disorder
- Uncapping and fenestration of cyst
  - o Hemiparesis improved in 30%
  - o Intractable seizures
    - Resolved in 62%
    - Improved in 24%
  - o No operative mortality

Selected References
1. Nowaczyk MJ et al: Antenatal and postnatal findings in encephalocraniocutaneous lipomatosis. Am J Med Genet 91:261-6, 2000
2. Koch CA et al: Fenestration of porencephalic cysts to the lateral ventricle: Experience with a new technique for treatment of seizures. Surg Neurol 49:524-32, 1998
3. Dildy GA et al: Porencephalic cyst: A complication of fetal intravascular transfusion. Am J Obstet Gynecol 165:76-8, 1991

Arachnoid Cyst

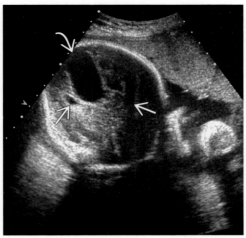

Arachnoid cyst. Sonographic image at the level of ventricles (arrows) shows a cystic lesion adjacent to the falx (curved arrow). Skull ossification causes considerable loss of intracranial detail in this third trimester fetus.

Key Facts
- Definition: CSF collection enclosed within layers of arachnoid
- Classic imaging appearance: Simple cyst displacing normal structures
- Nondestructive lesion which displaces normal structures
- Prenatal
  - 2/3 supratentorial
  - 1/3 infratentorial
- Postnatal majority in posterior fossa

Imaging Findings
General Features
- Best imaging clue: Extraaxial simple cyst
Ultrasound Findings
- Simple cyst
- Remaining brain sonographically normal in majority of cases
- Agenesis of corpus callosum in 5% with supratentorial arachnoid cyst (AC)
  - Absent cavum septi pellucidi
  - Colpocephaly
  - Stenogyria: Radiating narrow gyri medial surface of brain
  - Pericallosal artery: Absent/abnormal course
MR Findings
- SSFSE
  - Simple arachnoid cyst displaces normal parenchyma
  - Buckles gray/white matter interface
  - CSF signal
  - Look for associated findings
    - Agenesis of corpus callosum (5% with supratentorial AC)
    - Hydrocephalus

Arachnoid Cyst

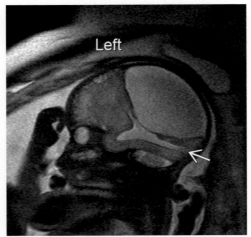

Arachnoid cyst. Fetal MRI. Sagittal SSFSE sequence shows cystic lesion displacing normal brain parenchyma. Compression of the left cerebral hemisphere and Foramen of Monro results in enlargement of the temporal horn (arrow). This cyst enlarged during pregnancy requiring postnatal shunt placement.

Differential Diagnosis
Porencephalic Cyst
- **Replaces damaged** brain
  - Arachnoid cyst **displaces normal** brain

Vein of Galen Aneurysm
- Midline
- Posterior
- Flow on Doppler

Schizencephaly
- Cleft in brain substance
- Lined with gray matter on MRI

Intracranial Hemorrhage
- May appear cystic if subacute
- Associated with destruction of normal tissue
- Blood products
  - High signal on FMPSPGR
  - Low signal on SSFSE
  - Arachnoid cyst follows CSF signal

Glioependymal Cyst
- Frontal or parietotemporal
- Centered on midline
  - Arachnoid cysts tend to extend to either side
- Protein content of cyst fluid higher
  - May alter signal in MRI allowing differentiation

Pathology
General
- General Path Comments
  - CSF containing cyst with thin membrane

Arachnoid Cyst

- Genetics
  - Mostly sporadic
  - Can be seen as part of syndromes
    - Neurofibromatosis Type 1
    - Multiple congenital anomaly disorders with single gene mutation
  - Trisomy 18
- Embryology
  - Frontal, temporal embryonic meninges (endomeninx) fail to merge as Sylvian fissure forms (middle cranial fossa)
  - Remain separate forming "duplicated" arachnoid
  - Older theory: Diverticulation of developing arachnoid
- Etiology-Pathogenesis
  - Possible mechanisms
    - Active fluid secretion by cyst wall
    - Slow distention by CSF pulsations
    - CSF accumulates by one-way (ball-valve) flow
- Epidemiology
  - Prenatal incidence unknown
  - 1% space-occupying lesions in childhood
  - 0.5% autopsies
  - M > F

Clinical Issues

Presentation
- Reported cases diagnosed in first trimester on endovaginal (EV) scan ultrasound

Natural History
- May cause hydrocephalus: More likely to occur with
  - Early gestational age at diagnosis
  - Size > 15 mm
  - Increasing size

Treatment
- Consider amniocentesis for karyotype even if isolated
- No prenatal intervention
- Monitor for growth of cyst
- Monitor for hydrocephalus
  - Head size may impact timing and mode of delivery

Prognosis
- Good if isolated abnormality
  - May require shunt or excision if mass effect
- Other anomalies determine prognosis when present

Selected References
1. Bannister C et al: Fetal arachnoid cysts: Their site, progress, prognosis, and differential diagnosis. Eur J Pediatr Surg 9:27-8, 1999
2. Barjot P et al: Diagnosis of arachnoid cysts on prenatal ultrasound. Fetal Diagn Ther 14:306-9, 1999
3. Hassan J et al: Glioependymal and arachnoid cysts: Unusual cause of early ventriculomegaly in utero. Prenat Diagn 16:729-33, 1996

Choroid Plexus Cyst

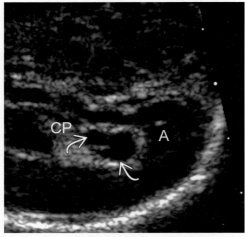

Choroid plexus cyst. Two small adjacent cysts (arrows) are seen in echogenic choroid plexus (CP) of left lateral ventricle. Notice the normal fluid filled atrium (A) separate and posterior to CP. In this case, choroid plexus cysts were an isolated finding and fetal outcome was normal.

Key Facts
- Definition: Cyst or cysts of fetal choroid plexus
- Classic imaging appearance: Sonolucent round cyst or cysts within choroid plexus in second trimester
- Seen in approximately **1% of all second trimester pregnancies**
- Choroid plexus cyst (CPC) is **marker for trisomy 18** (T18)
- Once detected, major challenge is decision about amniocentesis
  - Isolated finding vs associated markers/abnormalities
  - Low risk patient vs high risk patient
- CPC are benign transient finding
  - Not associated with adverse outcome in normal fetuses

Imaging Findings
General Features
- Best imaging clue: One or more round anechoic thick walled cysts seen in choroid plexus of lateral ventricles during second trimester
Ultrasound Findings
- CPC easily seen on routine lateral ventricle image
  - Transverse view of lateral ventricle at level of atria
  - Normal posterior **fluid-filled atria should not be confused with CPC**
    - Choroid is echogenic and fills body, not atria, of lateral ventricle
    - When CPC seen, oblique views confirm cyst is in choroid
  - Small cyst seen **surrounded by choroid**
- Diagnose cyst only when **diameter > 2 mm**
  - Choroid normally sponge-like
  - Tiny anechoic areas are not CPC
  - Look for discernable echogenic wall

Choroid Plexus Cyst

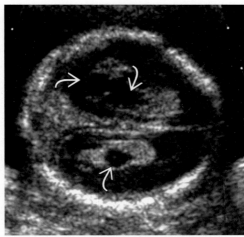

Choroid plexus cyst. Bilateral small choroid plexus cysts are seen (curved arrows). A "strawberry-shaped" calvarium is also present. The fetus had a cardiac anomaly, clenched hands with overlapping fingers, and clubfeet. Amniocentesis results revealed trisomy 18.

- Large CPC measure > 10 mm
  - o May be mistaken for ventriculomegaly
  - o More likely bilateral
  - o Increased association with chromosome abnormality
  - o Resolve slower
- **Multiple and bilateral CPC are common**
  - o Does not increase risk of chromosome abnormality
  - o Small cysts often seen in cluster
- Transient finding
  - o **All resolve in third trimester**
    - ▪ **Regardless of associated anomalies or isolated**
  - o Follow-up ultrasound to show resolution is not necessary

Imaging Recommendations
- **Determine if finding is isolated**
  - o Careful search for minor markers and major anomalies
- Search extremities for markers of T18
  - o Overlapping fingers
    - ▪ **Document open hands** in every case with CPC
  - o Clubfoot/rockerbottom foot
    - ▪ Document normal foot/leg relationship
- **Careful evaluation of fetal heart**
  - o Document normal outflow tracts

Differential Diagnosis
Lateral Ventricle Dilatation
- Large CPC may mimic distended lateral ventricle
- CPC surrounded by choroid while choroid "dangles" in large ventricle
Intraventricular Hemorrhage
- Rare in utero

Choroid Plexus Cyst

- Blood initially more echogenic than CPC
- Associated with hemorrhage at caudothalamic junction
- Blood present in ventricular regions usually free of choroid

Choroid Plexus Papilloma
- Rare tumor of choroid plexus
- Produces CSF
  - Associated hydrocephalus possible
- Papilloma usually hypoechoic while CPC are anechoic

Pathology

General
- General Path Comments
  - Choroid plexus normally located in body of lateral ventricle
  - Not in frontal, temporal, occipital horns
- Etiology-Pathogenesis
  - Not clear since CPC are transient
  - CPC play role in cerebral spinal fluid production
  - Cysts may be from trapped fluid
- Epidemiology
  - 1% of normal pregnancies
  - **50% of fetuses with T18**

Clinical Issues

Presentation
- Most commonly an **isolated finding in low-risk patient**
  - Isolated
    - No other minor markers or major anomalies
  - Low-risk patient
    - Not advanced maternal age
    - Normal maternal biochemical screen
- Sometimes: CPC + other fetal abnormalities

Natural History
- Transient finding, resolves in 3rd trimester
- Not associated with abnormal outcome in normal fetuses

Treatment
- None necessary for CPC

Prognosis
- Excellent prognosis for isolated CPC in low risk patient
  - Common, in 1% of all pregnancies on routine exam
  - Mildly increased risk for T18 but < 2x baseline risk
  - **Without other markers, not increased risk for trisomy 21 (T21)**
  - Amniocentesis not necessary
- Guarded prognosis for CPC + other abnormalities
  - CPC + minor markers = 20% risk for chromosome abnormality
  - CPC + major anomaly = 50% risk for chromosome abnormality
  - Amniocentesis warranted

Selected References
1. Ghidini A et al: Isolated fetal choroid plexus cysts: Role of ultrasonography in establishment of the risk of trisomy 18. Am J Obstet Gynecol 182:972-7, 2000
2. Gray DL et al: Is genetic amniocentesis warranted when isolated choroid plexus cysts are found? Prenat Diagn 16:983-90, 1996
3. Snijders RJ et al: Fetal choroid plexus cysts and trisomy 18: Assessment of risk based on ultrasound findings and maternal age. Prenat Diagn 14:1119-27, 1994

Intracranial Hemorrhage

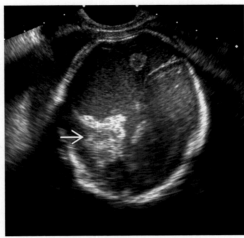

Intracranial hemorrhage. Endovaginal ultrasound of fetal head shows echogenic mass representing thrombus (arrow). Note the liquefaction of surrounding brain parenchyma with almost no recognizable structures visible.

Key Facts
- Definition: Bleeding within fetal cranium
- Classic imaging appearance: Echogenic foci in ventricles, parenchyma, or CSF spaces
- Classified as
  - Subdural/subarachnoid
  - Intraparenchymal
  - Periventricular: Graded same as germinal matrix hemorrhage (GMH)

Imaging Findings
General features
- Best imaging clue: Non-perfused, echogenic, intracranial "mass"
Ultrasound Findings
- Echogenic ependyma
- Hydrocephalus
- Subdural: Distance cortex to skull vault normally ≤ 4 mm
- Intraparenchymal ⇒ porencephaly
- Periventricular: Same appearance/grading as neonatal GMH
MR Findings
- SSFSE: Blood products low signal, confirm location on multiple planes
  - Do not confuse with flow artifact
    - Less defined signal: "Swirl" not mass-like
    - Location inconsistent sequence to sequence
- Septations in CSF spaces/ventricles correlate with hemorrhage and infection
- Blood/CSF levels
- Large flow voids: Feeding/draining vessels from vascular malformation
- Look for periventricular leukomalacia (PVL)/porencephaly

Intracranial Hemorrhage

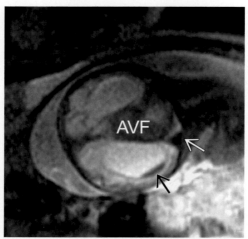

Intracranial hemorrhage. Fetal MRI. Coronal SSFSE image shows blood/CSF levels in the lateral ventricle (black arrow) and posterior fossa (white arrow). IVH occurred after thrombosis of a dural arteriovenous fistula (AVF). High signal in the surrounding white matter represented PVL (better seen on other sequences).

Imaging Recommendations
- Anemia secondary to hemorrhage increases risk for hydrops
  - Pericardial/pleural effusion
  - Ascites
  - Skin thickening
- **Use color Doppler**
- Peak systolic velocity in middle cerebral artery can be used to monitor anemia and need for intrauterine transfusion
- Thrombosis of vascular malformation ⇒ venous hypertension ⇒ bleed
  - Shape/location may suggest Vein of Galen aneurysm
  - Tubular components suggest thrombosed feeding/draining vessels

Differential Diagnosis
Intracranial Tumor
- Large, heterogeneous, rapidly growing
  - Clot will retract and decrease in echogenicity over time
- Perfused: Clot is avascular
- Macrocephaly: Space occupying lesion
  - ICH ⇒ parenchymal destruction ⇒ decreased head size
Infection
- Also causes destructive lesions and hydrops
  - Intracranial calcifications suggest CMV or Toxoplasmosis

Pathology
General
- General Path Comments
  - 6% of autopsies for stillbirth

Intracranial Hemorrhage

- Genetics
  - Alloimmune thrombocytopenia (AITP): Autosomal Dominant (AD)
  - Coagulation disorders: Some AD
  - Hemophilia: X-linked recessive
- Etiology-Pathogenesis
  - Alterations in maternal/fetal blood pressure
    - Seizure disorders
    - Drug use: Cocaine
    - Pre-eclamptic toxemia (PET)
    - Placental abruption
  - Trauma
    - Polynesian massage for external version of breech: Significant incidence of fetal subdural hematoma
    - Motor vehicle accident/domestic violence
  - Maternal thrombocytopenia/coagulation disorders
  - Hemorrhage-elevated liver function-low platelet (HELLP) syndrome
  - Fetal AVM/AVF
- Epidemiology
  - 1:1,000

Clinical Issues
Natural History
- Maternal idiopathic thrombocytopenia (ITP): Fetal ICH in < 1%
- AITP: Fetal ICH in 10-30%
Treatment
- Deliver by C-section
- Fetal transfusion: Platelets or whole blood
- AITP weekly infusion immune globulin +/- steroids
  - Good outcome in 8/8 infants
  - Prior to this therapy outcome was uniformly poor
Prognosis
- Increased incidence of
  - Seizure disorder
  - Cerebral palsy
  - Hydrocephalus
  - Developmental delay
- Outcome relates to severity and extent of bleed
- Poor outcome = demise or severe neurological impairment
  - In 88% subdural/subarachnoid bleeds
  - In 92% parenchymal bleeds
- Good outcome = normal or mild neurological impairment
- Periventricular bleed good outcome
  - In 100% Grade 1
  - In 60% Grade 2
  - In 0% Grade 3

Selected References
1. Sharif U et al: Prenatal intracranial hemorrhage and neurological complications in alloimmune thrombocytopenia. J Child Neurol 16:838-42, 2001
2. Green P et al: Idiopathic intracranial hemorrhage in the fetus. Fetal Diagn Ther 14:275-8, 1999
3. Vergani P et al: Clinical significance of fetal intracranial hemorrhage. Am J Obstet Gynecol 176:731-2, 1996

PocketRadiologist®
Obstetrics
Top 100 Diagnoses

FACE/NECK

Cleft Lip/Palate

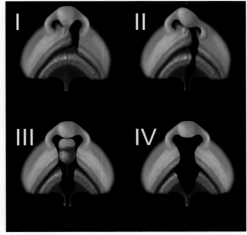

Cleft lip/palate. Ultrasound classification of four common types of cleft lip with and without cleft palate. Type 1: Unilateral cleft lip; type 2: Unilateral cleft lip with cleft palate; type 3: Bilateral cleft lip and palate; type 4: Midline cleft lip and palate.

Key Facts
- Synonyms: Cleft lip/palate (CL/P), facial cleft
- Definition: Congenital deformity resulting from unilateral or bilateral non-fusion of upper lip +/- associated non-fusion defect of palate
- Classic imaging appearance: **Lip skin line defect +/- defect of maxillary alveolar ridge**
- **Ultrasound classification**: 4 types of CL/P
  - Type 1: Unilateral cleft lip (CL) with intact palate
  - Type 2: Unilateral CL/P
  - Type 3: Bilateral CL/P
  - Type 4: Midline CL/P
- Cleft palate without CL involves more posterior soft palate
  - Difficult to diagnose in utero
- 20% type 1, 50% type 2-4, 30% cleft palate without CL
- **Associated with chromosome abnormalities and anomalies**
  - Predominately types 3 and 4

Imaging Findings
General Features
- Best imaging clue: Angled coronal ("**snout view**") shows linear or large defect of upper lip
- Profile views often abnormal, especially with large and bilateral CL/P
Ultrasound Findings
- Type 1
  - "Snout view": Linear defect of upper lip +/- nasal deformity
- Type 2
  - "Snout view": Similar to type 1, **nasal deformity** very likely
  - **Defect in palate seen best on axial/transverse view**
    - Amniotic fluid fills gap in alveolar ridge of maxilla

Cleft Lip/Palate

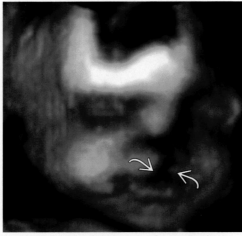

Cleft lip/palate. Three dimensional ultrasound surface rendered image of type 1 cleft lip (arrows).

- Type 3
  - o "Snout view": Very abnormal, bilateral lip defect, always nasal deformity
  - o Profile view: Mass-like **premaxillary protrusion**
    - ▪ "Island" of dysplastic anterior palate migrates forward
  - o Axial view: Bilateral lip and palate disruption seen best in this view
- Type 4
  - o Midline gap involving lip and palate
  - o Usually large and seen easily on all views
  - o Anterior midline hard palate is missing
- Isolated cleft palate: Rarely diagnosed in utero
  - o Posterior soft palate defect
- **Three dimensional ultrasound (3DUS)**
  - o Multiplanar images of CL/P most helpful tool of 3DUS
    - ▪ One acquisition can provide profile, axial, and "snout views"
    - ▪ Improves ability to evaluate extent of CL/P
  - o Surface rendered images: Lifelike pictures of fetal face
    - ▪ Psychologically prepares parents
  - o Helpful for plastic surgeons performing prenatal consultation
- Associated anomalies, syndromes, and chromosome abnormalities
  - o Structural anomalies in 14% type 1, 40% type 2-4 (most 3-4)
    - ▪ All organ system anomalies described
  - o Chromosome associations (patterns of anomalies help make diagnosis)
    - ▪ **Trisomy 13:** Type 4 most common
    - ▪ Trisomies 18, 22, 9, and 10
  - o Van der Woude syndrome: Autosomal dominant, 50% with CL/P

Imaging Recommendations
- Routine fetal snout and profile views
- Consider 3DUS for additional information

Cleft Lip/Palate

Differential Diagnosis
Amniotic Band Syndrome
- Amniotic bands cause **severe random "slash" defects**
- Clefts do not follow embryologic pattern
- Fetus may swallow disrupted bands

Normal Philtrum
- May resemble midline cleft defect on "snout view"
- Additional views show skin and palate intact
- Most prominent in large fetuses and late gestation

Facial Mass (Anterior Cephalocele, Epignathus, Facial Hemangioma)
- May resemble premaxillary protrusion of type 3 CL/P
- Look for secondary changes in brain (cephalocele)
- Intact palate with hemangioma
- **Epignathus (teratoma)**: Large, bizarre mass from nose and mouth

Pathology
General
- Etiology-Pathogenesis
  o Embryology
    ▪ CL: Failure of normal fusion of 3 lip segments (2 lateral, 1 middle)
    ▪ CL/P: CL + failure of normal fusion of 3 primary palate segments
    ▪ CP alone: Failure of normal fusion of 2 secondary palate segments
- Epidemiology
  o 0.15% of all births, 7.5% of all anomalies
  o CL/P: **1:600 Asian**, 1:1,000 Caucasian, 1:2,500 African-American
  o Isolated cleft palate rate is same for all ethnic groups
  o Males more common for CL/P, females for isolated CP
  o Unilateral CL/P more common on left
  o Chromosome abnormalities and CL/P
    ▪ Rare for type 1, 20% for 2, 30% for 3, 52% for 4

Clinical Issues
Presentation
- **Polyhydramnios** when severe and interferes with swallowing
- Incidentally noted on screening prenatal exam

Treatment
- **Amniocentesis should be considered for types 2-4**
- Sometimes repaired immediately after birth
- Cleft lip usually repaired few months after birth
- Cleft palate usually repaired at 9-18 months

Prognosis
- Depends on associated anomalies and chromosome results
- Multiple surgeries may be needed
- Speech therapy, dental procedures may be necessary
- Associated ear/nose/throat problems

Selected References
1. Clementi M et al: Evaluation of prenatal diagnosis of cleft lip with or without cleft palate and cleft palate by ultrasound. Prenat Diagn 20:870-5, 2000
2. Nyberg DA et al: Fetal cleft lip with and without cleft palate: US classification and correlation with outcome. Radiology 195:677-83, 1995
3. Benacerraf BR et al: Fetal cleft lip/palate: Sonographic diagnosis and postnatal outcome. Plast Reconstr Surg 92:1045-51, 1993

Micrognathia

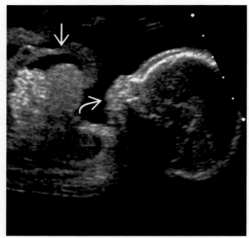

Micrognathia. Ultrasound image of a fetus with trisomy 18. Note the receding chin and lower lip (curved arrow). There is also an omphalocele containing liver and bowel (arrow).

Key Facts
- Definition: Small mandible
  - Receding chin
  - Abnormal posterior position of tongue: Glossoptosis
- Classic imaging appearance: Receding chin on profile view
- Micrognathia is a component of over 70 named syndromes
- Most important question: **What else is abnormal**
- Subgroups of conditions featuring micrognathia
  - Chromosome/single gene disorders
    - Trisomy 18, 13, 9, 8
    - Treacher Collins
    - Stickler syndrome
    - Smith-Lemli-Opitz
  - Named syndromes
    - Pierre Robin
  - Neuromuscular/skeletal disorders
    - Fetal akinesia sequence
    - Neu-Lavoxa syndrome
  - Teratogen exposure
    - Valproic acid
    - Methotrexate

Imaging Findings
General Features
- Best imaging clue: Receding chin on **true sagittal** image of face
Ultrasound Findings
- 3D US may be best method to evaluate facial structures
  - Volumetric acquisition
  - Ensure accurate sagittal section

Micrognathia

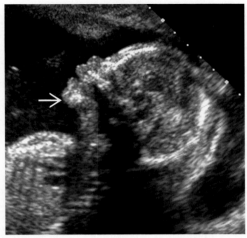

Normal fetal profile for comparison to micrognathia. Sagittal sonogram shows the mandible (arrow) covered by the soft tissues of the chin. Mandible and maxilla are at approximately the same level as the forehead.

- Jaw index
  - AP diameter mandible/BPD x 100
- Polyhydramnios: Associated in up to 70%
  - Abnormal swallowing
- Strong association with
  - Skeletal dysplasia
  - Congenital heart disease
  - Cystic hygroma
  - Intrauterine growth restriction
- Other associated anomalies
  - Tracheo-esophageal fistula

MR Findings
- Single shot FSE imaging used to assess
  - Cleft palate
  - CNS anomalies

Imaging Recommendations
- Care to image profile in true sagittal plane, if off axis may "create" receding jaw
- Axial section through toothbuds in maxilla for associated cleft palate
- Use 3D if available
- Fetal ears
  - Treacher Collins: Small ears may not be visible
  - Nager syndrome: Malformed ears, poorly ossified upper extremity bones
  - Goldenhar syndrome: Malformed ear, hemifacial microsomia
  - Otocephaly: Hypoplasia or absence of mandible associated with
    - Synotia: Ventromedial displacement external ears to midline neck
    - Microstomia, aglossia, nose-mouth fusion

Micrognathia

- Fetal eyes
  - Neu-Lavoxa: Hypertelorism, protruding eyes, absent eyelids

Differential Diagnosis
Agnathia
- Absent mandible
- Lethal

Pathology
General
- Genetics
  - Autosomal dominant
    - Treacher Collins
    - Stickler syndrome
  - Autosomal recessive
    - Smith-Lemli-Opitz
    - Neu-Lavoxa
  - Many cases are new spontaneous mutations
- Epidemiology: Incidence unknown-heterogeneous group of conditions
  - Pierre Robin 1:30,000
  - Trisomy 18 1:3,000 live births

Clinical Issues
Presentation
- Significant mandibular growth occurs in third trimester $\Rightarrow$ severity may not be apparent at 18 to 20 week scan
Treatment
- Genetic counseling
  - Detailed family history
  - Teratogen exposure
- Offer karyotype: 66% abnormal chromosomes
- Deliver at tertiary center
  - Airway difficulties at birth
  - Feeding problems
  - Sleep-related airway obstruction
Prognosis
- Prenatal diagnosis
  - 30% termination
  - 50% intrauterine or early neonatal demise
- Recurrence risk
  - Autosomal dominant 50%
  - Autosomal recessive 25%
  - Aneuploidy 1% or maternal age related

Selected References
1. Paladini D et al: Objective diagnosis of micrognathia in the fetus: the jaw index. Obstet Gynecol 93:382-6, 1999
2. Cohen J et al: Prenatal sonographic diagnosis of Treacher Collins syndrome: A case and review of the literature. Am J Perinatol 12:416-9, 1995
3. King JA et al: Neu-Lavoxa syndrome: Pathological evaluation of a fetus and review of the literature. Pediatr Pathol Lab Med 15:57-9, 1995

Epignathus

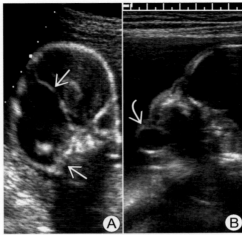

Epignathus. (A) Coronal sonogram of the fetal head shows a mixed cystic/solid mass centered at the skull base with both intracranial and pharyngeal extension (arrows). (B) Sagittal image shows extension of this mass through the fetal mouth (curved arrow).

Key Facts
- Synonym: Nasopharyngeal teratoma, oral teratoma, facial teratoma
- Definition: Teratoma arising in oral cavity or pharynx
- Classic imaging appearance: Complex, mixed cystic/solid mass emanating from mouth or nose
- Begins in region of palate or basisphenoid
  - Preferential growth into nasopharynx, oropharynx, and out mouth or nose
  - May extend intracranially with distortion of brain
- **Benign by histology, often lethal by location**
- Nasopharyngeal/facial location < 2%
- More common in other areas
  - Sacrococcygeal 50-60%
  - Chest/abdomen 15-35%
  - Brain < 5%

Imaging Findings
General Features
- Best imaging clue: **Calcification** helps differentiate from other masses in this region
- Fills oral cavity and emanates from mouth and/or nose
- **May extend up into cranium as an extra-axial mass**
  - Can cause marked distortion of intracranial structures
Ultrasound Findings
- Predominately solid or mixed cystic/solid
- Can be massive
- Hypertelorism
- Exophthalmos
- Splayed mandible
- Cervical hyperextension

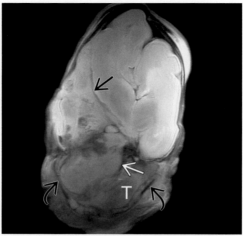

Epignathus. Postmortem T2WI of the same fetus shows both pharyngeal (white arrow) and intracranial extension of the mass (black arrow). The intracranial portion is causing significant extra-axial mass effect on the brain. The mandible is splayed (curved arrows) with deviation of the tongue (T).

- **Polyhydramnios** secondary to pharyngeal obstruction
- Hydrops late finding with large masses
  - High output cardiac failure
- Cardiac anomalies may be associated

MR Findings
- Helpful in determining anatomic extent
- Can identify fat within lesion
- Rules out anterior cephalocele

Imaging Recommendations
- Routine head and face views should detect virtually all cases
- Color Doppler to evaluate vascularity
- Close interval scanning
  - **May grow rapidly to massive size**
    - Often larger than fetal head
  - May extend intracranially
    - Compresses and displaces normal brain parenchyma
    - Head enlargement
    - Hydrocephalus
  - Worsening polyhydramnios

Differential Diagnosis

Anterior Cephalocele
- Direct continuity with brain
- Distortion of intracranial anatomy
- **MRI** confirms diagnosis

Cervical Teratoma
- Mass arises from anterior neck below mandible
- No intraoral or intracranial extension
- May extend into mediastinum

Epignathus

- May be difficult to tell point of origin with large masses

Cystic Hygroma
- Posterior neck mass
- Mouth, pharynx, and brain normal
- Cystic with septations
- No calcification

Pathology

General
- Genetics
  - o Sporadic
- Embryology
  - o Abnormal migration of primordial germ cells
- Epidemiology
  - o Rare

Microscopic Features
- Germ cell tumor containing at least one of three germ cell layers
  - o Often contains nerve tissue ("brain-like")
  - o Fat, cartilage, and bone
- Majority histologically benign

Clinical Issues

Presentation
- Reported as early as 15 weeks
- Polyhydramnios

Natural History
- May show rapid in utero growth

Treatment
- Termination offered
- If pregnancy continued deliver at tertiary care facility
- Large masses may cause dystocia
  - o Cesarean section be necessary
- Plan for immediate tracheostomy for ventilation

Prognosis
- Generally fatal but surgical techniques improving
- No recurrence risk

Selected References
1. Papageorgiou C et al: Prenatal diagnosis of epignathus in the first half of pregnancy: A case report and review of the literature. Clin Exp Obstet Gynecol 27:67-8, 2000
2. Gull I et al: Antenatal sonographic diagnosis of epignathus at 15 weeks of pregnancy. Ultrasound Obstet Gynecol 13:271-3, 1999
3. McMahon MJ et al: Perinatal management of a lingual teratoma. Obstet Gynecol 87:848-51, 1996

Cystic Hygroma

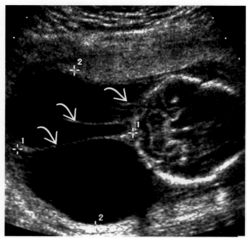

Cystic hygroma. Large cystic hygroma (calipers) in a second trimester fetus with Turner syndrome. Note the septations in the subcutaneous fluid (curved arrows).

Key Facts
- Synonyms: Lymphangioma, nuchal cystic hygromata
- Definition: Congenital abnormality of lymphatic vessels leading to cysts in subcutaneous tissue
  - Most common location in fetal life is behind neck
- Classic imaging appearance: Large **septated fluid collections** involving skin behind fetal neck
- **Nuchal** cystic hygroma (CH)
  - Considered a major marker for chromosome aneuploidy
  - **Chromosome abnormalities in 2/3** of cases
    - **Turner syndrome** (X0) most common
  - Associated with **hydrops** fetalis in 40%
- Part of spectrum of increased nuchal translucency seen in 1st trimester
- Non-nuchal CH uncommon and considered sporadic

Imaging Findings
General Features
- Best imaging clue: Subcutaneous fluid collections that are **mass-like** and usually located in posterior and lateral fetal neck
Ultrasound Findings
- Fluid masses involve skin and subcutaneous tissues
- Most commonly nuchal, seen behind and lateral to fetal neck
- Size varies but usually large
  - **Can mimic amniotic fluid** when oligohydramnios is present
  - Smaller collections may resolve
  - May become nuchal fold skin thickening with time
- Usually septated but can be simple
- Associated with other anomalies
  - Cardiac defects
  - Hydrops fetalis
    - Skin edema, ascites, pleural effusion, pericardial effusion

Cystic Hygroma

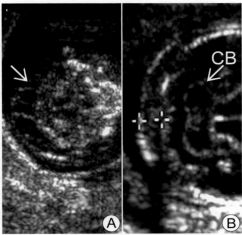

Cystic hygroma. (A, B) First trimester septated cystic hygroma (arrow) becomes nuchal fold thickening in the second trimester (calipers) in this fetus with Down syndrome (Trisomy 21). (CB - normal cerebellum).

Imaging Recommendations
- Look carefully for other anomalies
- Look for hydrops
- Follow up frequently
  - Increased incidence of in utero demise
  - May detect further anomalies as fetus grows (especially cardiac)

Differential Diagnosis

Occipital Encephalocele
- Variable amount of posterior fossa contents displaced through a visible cranial defect
  - Nuchal CH has **no cranial defect**

Hemangioma
- Vascular hamartoma seen in skin of head and neck
  - More solid than CH
  - May be able to show blood flow with color Doppler

Amniotic Band Syndrome
- Disruption of amnion leads to entrapment of fetal parts
  - Lymphedema: Not as cystic as CH
  - Limb amputation (usually fingers and toes)
  - Cleft defects in body and face (more asymmetric than with CH)

Pathology

General
- Etiology-Pathogenesis
  - Congenital abnormalities of lymphatics
  - Nuchal CH
    - Failed or delayed communication between internal jugular veins and jugular lymphatic sacs

Cystic Hygroma

- - Normal communication usually established 40 days from conception
- Epidemiology
  - o Nuchal CH associated with chromosome abnormalities in 2/3
    - Turner syndrome (X0)
    - Down syndrome (Trisomy 21)
    - Edwards syndrome (Trisomy 18)
  - o Nuchal CH associated with many non-karyotypic abnormalities
    - Noonan syndrome
    - Apert syndrome
    - Cornelia de Lange syndrome

Clinical Issues

Presentation
- Incidentally seen during routine second trimester ultrasound exam
- May be seen as increased nuchal translucency in first trimester exam
  - o Usually septated even in first trimester
- Found when looking for cause of nonimmune hydrops fetalis
- May be noted in cases of fetal demise

Treatment
- Amniocentesis for karyotyping
- Genetic counseling

Prognosis
- Septated CH associated with worse prognosis than nonseptated
  - o Higher incidence of aneuploidy and hydrops
- Depends on presence or absence of other anomalies
- Depends on chromosome results
- Grim prognosis if hydrops is present
- May result in thickened nuchal skin as gestation progresses
- Non-nuchal CH prognosis dependent upon surgical removal

Selected References
1. Reynders CS et al: First trimester isolated fetal nuchal lucency: Significance and outcome. J Ultrasound Med 16:101-5, 1997
2. Bronshtein M et al: The difference between septated and nonsepatated nuchal cystsic hygroma in the early second trimester. Obstet Gynecol 81:683-7, 1993
3. Thomas RL: Prenatal diagnosis of giant cystic hygroma. Prenatal Diagn 12:919-23, 1992

Goiter

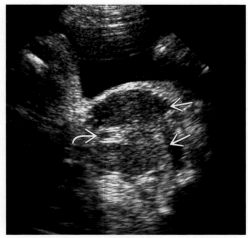

Goiter. Coronal section of fetal neck showing uniform enlargement of the thyroid lobes (arrows). The trachea (curved arrow) contains fluid therefore is not completely compressed.

Key Facts
- Definition: Enlargement of fetal thyroid
- Classic imaging appearance: Homogeneously echogenic neck mass
- **Goiter occurs with increased and decreased fetal thyroid function**
- Fetal thyroid status does not follow maternal
- Mass effect ⇒ neck extension ⇒ obstructed labor
- Large goiter may cause life-threatening airway obstruction at delivery
- Placental transfer throughout pregnancy
  - o Thyroid stimulating immunoglobulins (TSI)
  - o Thyrotropin releasing hormone (TRH)
  - o Antithyroid medication
  - o Iodides
  - o Beta blockers
- Decreasing placental transfer as pregnancy progresses
  - o Thyroid stimulating hormone (TSH)
  - o Triiodothyronine (T3)
  - o Thyroxine (T4)
- Fetal thyroid fully sensitive to TSI, antithyroid drugs by 20 weeks

Imaging Findings
<u>General Features</u>
- Best imaging clue: **Homogenous** neck mass
<u>Ultrasound Findings</u>
- Neck mass: **Maintains thyroid contour**
  - o Nomograms available for size at given gestational age
- Mass effect
  - o Obstructed swallowing ⇒ polyhydramnios
- Hydrops
  - o Vascular shunts ⇒ high output state
    - ▪ **Occurs in hyper- and hypothyroidism**

Goiter

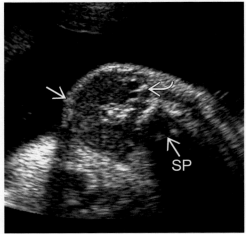

Goiter. Axial scan through fetal neck. The isthmus is thickened (arrow.). The jugular vein and carotid artery are also noted (curved arrow). SP - cervical spine.

- Growth disturbance
- Hyperthyroid
  - Fetal tachycardia
  - Craniosynostosis

MR Findings
- FMPSPGR
  - **Uniform high signal** due to iodine content
- SSFSE
  - Intermediate signal
  - Strap muscles low signal
  - Allows evaluation of tracheal and esophageal compression

Imaging Recommendations
- Monitor for
  - Growth
  - Heart rate and rhythm
  - Hydrops
  - Amniotic fluid volume
- Use color Doppler for thyroid vascularity

Differential Diagnosis
Cervical Teratoma
- Often very large, irregular shape
- Mixed echogenicity +/- calcifications

Pathology
General
- Etiology-Pathogenesis
  - Hyperthyroid
    - Transplacental maternal thyroid stimulating antibodies
  - Hypothyroid

Goiter

- Transplacental maternal anti-thyroid drugs
- Iodine insufficiency
- Genetics
  o Not hereditary
- Epidemiology
  o Rare, true incidence unknown
  o Iodine deficient areas: Pregnancy stresses maternal thyroid
    - Increased risk fetal hypothyroidism
  o 2-12% abnormal fetal thyroid function in mothers with Graves disease (autoimmune hyperthyroidism)

Clinical Issues
Presentation
- High index of suspicion with maternal history of Graves disease
- May present as neck mass despite maternal euthyroid state
Natural History
- Maternal Graves disease with persistent hyperthyroidism in pregnancy
  o Increased incidence miscarriage and stillbirth
- **Fetal hypothyroidism**
  o Studies suggest deficient myelination ⇒ learning difficulties
  o Unlikely to result in cretinism as neonatal treatment alone effective in prevention
- **Fetal hyperthyroidism**
  o Tachycardia ⇒ hydrops
Treatment
- Monitor maternal thyroid status with free T3, free T4
  o Thyroxine binding globulin increased in pregnancy
  o Spurious elevation of total T3, T4 in euthyroid pregnancy
- Check maternal thyroid antibody status if not known
- Cordocentesis for fetal free T3, free T4, and TSH levels
  o Normal ranges established
  o Fetal serum levels more reliable than amniotic fluid levels
- Fetal hypothyroidism
  o Weekly intra-amniotic injection of thyroxine
- Fetal hyperthyroidism
  o Maternal medication until fetal response
    - Propylthiouracil preferred
  o Thyroxine replacement as needed to keep mother euthyroid
- If persistent goiter consider EXIT procedure (**Ex** utero **Intrapartum Treatment**) for delivery
  o Infant maintained on placental support while airway is established
Prognosis
- Generally rapid response to treatment reported with
  o Reduction in size of goiter
  o Resolution polyhydramnios

Selected References
1. Agrawal P: Intrauterine diagnosis and management of congenital goitrous hypothyroidism. Ultrasound Obstet Gynecol 19:501-5, 2002
2. Gruner C et al: Intrauterine treatment of fetal goitrous hyperthyroidism controlled by determination of thyroid-stimulating hormone in fetal serum. A case report and review of the literature. Fetal Diagn Ther 16:47-51, 2001
3. Guibourdenche J et al: Biochemical investigation of foetal and neonatal thyroid function using the ACS-180SE analyzer. Ann Clin Biochem 38:520-6, 2001

Nuchal Cord

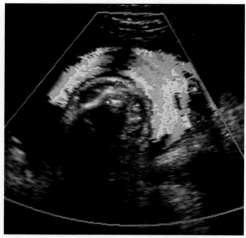

Nuchal cord. Transverse color Doppler image shows multiple loops of umbilical cord wrapped around the fetal neck. Four complete loops were noted at delivery.

Key Facts
- Definition: One or more complete loops of umbilical cord around fetal neck
- Classic imaging appearance: Cystic mass around neck which has **flow on color Doppler**
- Frequency increases with increasing gestational age
  - 6% at 20 weeks
  - 29% at 42 weeks
- May spontaneously unwind
- Multiple loops and evidence of pressure effects at greater risk for complications

Imaging Findings
General Features
- Best imaging clue: **Must see in both sagittal and transverse planes** to rule out false positive
Ultrasound Findings
- Compression effects on fetal skin **(divot sign)**
- Use color Doppler if cord seen near neck
  - Confirm diagnosis
  - Avoid missing nuchal cord not suspected in gray-scale
Imaging Recommendations
- Look for vascular compromise
  - Increased systolic to diastolic (S/D) ratio
  - Early diastolic notching
  - If umbilical artery abnormal interrogate middle cerebral artery
- Follow-up US with attention to
  - Growth
  - Amniotic fluid
    - Oligohydramnios increases risk of complication
  - Doppler flow

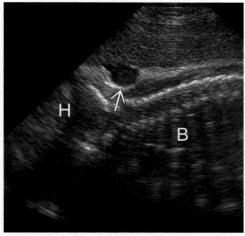

Nuchal cord with a divot sign in a fetus with oligohydramnios. Sagittal ultrasound image shows a single loop of umbilical cord wrapped around the back of the fetal neck (cord made a complete loop encircling the neck). Note the prominent skin impression (divot sign - arrow). (H - head, B - body).

- o Fetal movement
- 3D ultrasound may aid in evaluation

Differential Diagnosis
<u>Cord Adjacent to Neck</u>
- Will not form complete loop around neck
  - o Not present in both sagittal and transverse
- Will change during course of exam or on follow-up
<u>Cystic Hygroma</u>
- Multiseptated mass
- No Doppler flow

Pathology
<u>General</u>
- Etiology-Pathogenesis (proposed)
  - o Cords with less vascular coiling are more pliable and at greater risk
  - o Longer cords at increased risk
- Epidemiology
  - o Prevalence 8-30%
  - o More common in males
    - ▪ Longer cords
<u>Gross Pathologic, Surgical Features</u>
- Type A
  - o Umbilical end of cord passes over the placental end
  - o Can spontaneously unwind
- Type B
  - o Umbilical end of cord passes under the placental end
  - o "Locking" type
  - o Greater risk for stillbirth

Nuchal Cord

o May move down cord to form knot

Clinical Issues
Presentation
- Incidental finding
Natural History
- Vast majority of no consequence
- Reported associations (usually not associated with long-term sequelae)
  o Growth restriction
  o Intrapartum fetal distress
  o Low Apgar scores
  o Meconium staining
  o Lower umbilical artery pH
  o Assisted ventilation (< 30 min)
- Rare serious complications
  o Developmental delay
  o Spastic quadriplegia
  o Stillbirth
- **Risk increases with**
  o **Tightness**
  o **Multiple loops**
  o **Oligohydramnios**
Treatment
- **Always include in report**
- Patient should be made aware of importance of decreased fetal movement
- Consider non-stress test (NST) and biophysical profile if any concerns arise
- Early delivery for deteriorating status
- Most reduced during delivery without consequence
Prognosis
- Excellent

Selected References
1. Callen PW: Categorical Course in Diagnostic Radiology: The umbilical cord looks funny: What does that mean? RSNA, Chicago. 9-20, 2002
2. Sherer DM et al: Prenatal ultrasonographic diagnosis of nuchal cord(s): Disregard, inform, monitor, or intervene? Ultrasound Obstet Gynecol 14:1-8, 1999
3. Collins JH: Nuchal cord type A and type B. Am J Obstet Gynecol 177:94, 1997

PocketRadiologist®
Obstetrics
Top 100 Diagnoses

CHEST

Cystic Adenomatoid Malformation

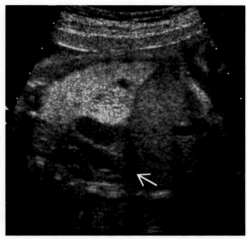

Cystic adenomatoid malformation. Coronal sonogram of the fetal chest shows a markedly hyperechoic mass filling the left hemithorax and displacing the heart to the right (arrow).

Key Facts
- Synonym: Congenital cystic adenomatoid malformation (CCAM)
- Definition: Lung hamartoma with proliferation of terminal bronchioles and lack of normal alveoli
- Classic imaging appearance: Unilateral solid or mixed cystic/solid chest mass
- **Most common** fetal lung mass (75%)
- Communicates with tracheobronchial tree
- **May spontaneously regress**
- Development of hydrops is dismal prognosis
  - o Occurs in less than 10% of cases
- No side predilection

Imaging Findings
General Features
- Best imaging clue: Solid or cystic lung mass with **arterial supply from pulmonary artery**
- 95% are unilateral and affect only 1 lobe
- Other anomalies in 3-12%
Ultrasound Findings
- Sonographic classification (variation of pathologic classification below)
  - o Macrocystic: 1 or more cysts 5 mm or greater
  - o Microcystic: Homogeneously echogenic, cysts < 5 mm
- Stomach will be in normal location
Imaging Recommendations
- Use color Doppler to identify feeding vessel
- Monitor closely (every 1-2 weeks) after initial diagnosis for growth, development of hydrops, or polyhydramnios
- If regression or no change, can increase time interval between scans
- Fetal echo suggested

Cystic Adenomatoid Malformation

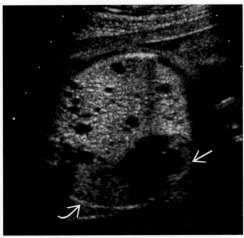

Cystic adenomatoid malformation. An axial image in the same fetus shows several macroscopic cysts within the echogenic mass. Note the compressed contralateral lung (curved arrow) and displacement of the heart (arrow).

Differential Diagnosis

Extralobar Sequestration (ELS)
- **Feeding vessel from aorta**
- Uniformly echogenic
- 90% left-sided

Congenital Diaphragmatic Hernia
- Absent normal fluid-filled stomach
- Abdominal circumference small
- **Peristalsis** is pathognomonic
- Other anomalies common

Hybrid Lesion (CCAM + ELS)
- Histology shows both lesions
- Consider when there is a systemic vessel feeding a cystic lung mass

Congenital Lobar Emphysema
- Uniformly echogenic
- More commonly upper lobe
- Rare to diagnose in utero

Tracheal Atresia
- May be confused for bilateral CCAM
- Lungs are symmetrically enlarged (often grossly) and echogenic
- Fluid in the trachea and bronchi

Other Cystic Masses
- Bronchogenic cyst, neurenteric cyst, esophageal duplication cyst
- All rare
- More often associated with mediastinum

Pathology

General
- Genetics
  - o Sporadic inheritance

Cystic Adenomatoid Malformation

  o No recurrence risk
- Epidemiology
  o Considered rare but true incidence not known
  o Likely more common than previously thought

Pathologic Staging
- CCAM I: Cysts 2-10 cm
- CCAM II: Cysts < 2 cm
- CCAM III: Cysts < 0.5 cm

Clinical Issues
Presentation
- Usually an incidental finding

Natural History
- Wide spectrum of outcomes
- Majority remain stable or regress in utero
- Some may progress increasing risk of hydrops and death
- Postnatally at risk for infection
- **Small risk for developing malignancy**: Rhabdomyosarcoma, myxosarcoma, and bronchoalveolar carcinoma

Treatment
- None unless hydropic
- Hydrops > 32 weeks
  o Maternal betamethasone administration and early delivery
  o Immediate resection
- Hydrops < 32 weeks: In utero therapy
  o Macroscopic CCAM
    ▪ Cyst drainage: Temporizing measure only, fluid will recur
    ▪ Thoracoamniotic shunt
  o Microscopic CCAM
    ▪ In utero resection
- Delivery at a tertiary care facility
  o At risk for neonatal complications including air trapping and pneumothorax
- Postnatal workup of all lesions **even if regressed in utero**
  o Chest X-ray may not show lesion
  o CT or MRI may be necessary
- Postnatal resection somewhat controversial
  o Most feel small risk of malignancy warrants resection in all cases

Prognosis
- Dependent on mass size, degree of pulmonary hypoplasia, polyhydramnios, and hydrops
  o **100% mortality with hydrops** if untreated
- Excellent for small or spontaneously regressed masses

Selected References
1. Coleman BG et al: Fetal therapy: State of the art. J Ultrasound Med 21:1257-88, 2002
2. Adzick NS et al: Fetal lung lesions: Management and outcome. Am J Obstet Gynecol 179:884-9, 1998
3. Thorpe-Beeston JG et al: Cystic adenomatoid malformation of the lung: Prenatal diagnosis and outcome. Prenat Diagn 14:677-88, 1994

Sequestration

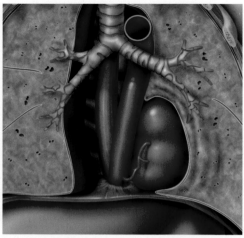

Extralobar sequestration. Illustration shows a sequestered lung segment in the left lung base covered with its own pleural investment. The vascular supply is from the aorta.

Key Facts
- Synonyms: Bronchopulmonary sequestration, Rokitansky lobe
- Definition: Bronchopulmonary tissue that does not connect to tracheobronchial tree or pulmonary arteries
  - Occurs in extralobar and intralobar forms
- Classic imaging appearance: Well-defined, homogeneously echogenic mass in left lower lobe
- **Extralobar sequestration (ELS)** vast majority of those seen in utero
- May spontaneously regress
- 5–10% develop **tension hydrothorax**
- **90% are left-sided**
- Up to 10% are below diaphragm
  - May be confused for an adrenal mass

Imaging Findings
General Features
- Best imaging clue: Solid lung mass with **arterial supply from aorta**
- Draining vein often difficult to visualize
- Presence of an associated **pleural effusion is highly suggestive of ELS**
- **Other anomalies in 10-50%**
  - Congenital diaphragmatic hernia most common
  - Cardiac malformations
  - Gastrointestinal
    - Tracheoesophageal fistula
    - Duplication cysts
Ultrasound Findings
- Homogeneously echogenic
- Well-defined triangular or lobar shape
- Typically left lower lobe

Sequestration

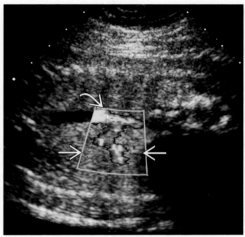

Extralobar sequestration. Coronal sonogram of the fetal chest with power Doppler shows a large feeding artery arising from the aorta (curved arrow) supplying the wedge-shaped echogenic lung mass (between two arrows).

Imaging Recommendations
- Use **color Doppler to identify feeding vessel**

Differential Diagnosis
Congenital Cystic Adenomatoid Malformation (CCAM)
- Microcystic type
- Feeding vessel from the **pulmonary artery**
- May occur on either side
Hybrid Lesion (CCAM + ELS)
- Histology shows both lesions
- Consider when there is a systemic vessel feeding a cystic lung mass
Congenital Lobar Emphysema
- Uniformly echogenic
- More commonly upper lobe
- Rare to diagnose in utero

Pathology
General
- Genetics
  - o   Sporadic inheritance
- Embryology
  - o   Ectopic budding of tracheobronchial tree
- Epidemiology
  - o   1:1,000 general population
  - o   Incidence in utero not known
  - o   Likely more common than previously thought
  - o   M:F = 4:1
Pathologic Types
- Extralobar
  - o   Own pleural investment

- o Drains to a systemic vessel
- o Histology
  - ▪ Dilated bronchioles and alveoli
  - ▪ Ectatic dilated lymphatics prominent feature
- Intralobar
  - o No pleural investment
  - o Drains to pulmonary vein
  - o May be acquired
    - ▪ Rare in utero or infancy
    - ▪ > 50% present over 20 years of age
    - ▪ May result from recurrent infection
    - ▪ Normal blood supply may be compromised with parasitization of systemic vessels
  - o Histology
    - ▪ Chronic inflammation and fibrosis

Clinical Issues
Presentation
- Usually an incidental finding
Natural History
- **50-75% will regress** in utero
- May be complicated by a tension hydrothorax
  - o Proposed mechanism
    - ▪ Leakage from ectatic lymphatics
    - ▪ Torsion of sequestered segment
  - o May progress to generalized hydrops from cardiovascular compression
- Postnatal
  - o Most are asymptomatic
  - o May have respiratory distress or cyanosis
  - o May present with associated abnormality
Treatment
- Drainage or thoracoamniotic shunt for tension hydrothorax
- Postnatal resection for persistent or symptomatic masses
- Resection may not be necessary for regressed lesions in asymptomatic individuals
Prognosis
- Excellent when a solitary finding even if complicated by hydrothorax or hydrops
- Poorer prognosis determined by associated abnormalities

Selected References
1. Goldstein RB: Categorical course in diagnostic radiology: Findings at US – what do they mean. RSNA, Chicago. 167-78, 2002
2. Lopoo JB et al: Fetal pulmonary sequestration: A favorable congenital lung lesion. Obstet Gynecol 94:567-71, 1999
3. Adzick NS et al: Fetal lung lesions: Management and outcome. Am J Obstet Gynecol 179:884-9, 1998

Congenital Diaphragmatic Hernia

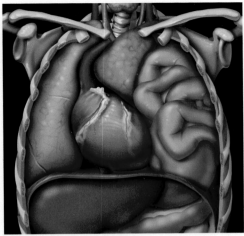

Congenital diaphragmatic hernia. Illustration shows posterior defect in the left hemidiaphragm with herniation of the stomach and small bowel into the left hemithorax. There is rightward mediastinal shift and compression of both the ipsilateral and contralateral lung.

Key Facts
- Definition: Herniation of abdominal contents into chest typically via posterior defect in diaphragm (foramen of Bochdalek)
- Classic imaging appearance: Cystic mass (bowel and stomach) within fetal thorax with deviation of heart to right
- 85-90% are left-sided
  - Remainder are either right-sided, bilateral, or retrosternal through foramen of Morgagni
- **Up to 50%** of congenital diaphragmatic hernias (CDH) will have an **associated abnormality**

Imaging Findings
General Features
- Best imaging clue: **Peristalsis within cystic chest mass is pathognomonic**
- Normal cardiac axis on four-chamber view rules out a significant CDH
- Abdominal circumference will measure less than expected

Ultrasound Findings
- Four findings of left-sided hernia
  - Cystic mass in left side of chest
  - Deviation of heart toward right
  - Absence of fluid-filled stomach
  - Polyhydramnios
- Right-sided more difficult: Lung and liver echogenecity is similar
  - Deviation of heart toward left
  - **Color Doppler helpful to trace portal vessels** into chest
  - Fetal stomach shifted toward midline

CT Findings
- Rarely used in obese patients
- Fetus will swallow contrast injected into amniotic fluid

Congenital Diaphragmatic Hernia

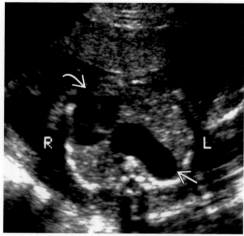

Congenital diaphragmatic hernia. Axial sonographic image of the fetal chest shows the stomach within the thoracic cavity (arrow) with displacement of the heart to the right (curved arrow).

MR Findings
- Coronal and sagittal planes most helpful for showing the defect
- Bowel appears as tubular serpiginous structures with variable signal intensity on both T1WI and T2WI
- Accurately diagnoses presence of liver in CDH ("liver-up")
  - Up to 85% of left-sided hernias have "liver-up"
- Can perform direct volumetric lung measurements

Imaging Recommendations
- All fetuses with CDH need dedicated fetal echo
  - CDH and cardiac defect is considered lethal
- Calculate a **lung-to-head ratio (LHR)**: Area of contralateral lung divided by head circumference
  - Lung area is calculated by multiplying 2 cross-sectional lung measurements taken at level of four-chamber view
  - LHR > 1.4 good prognosis
  - LHR < 1.0 poor prognosis

Differential Diagnosis

Congenital Cystic Adenomatoid Malformation (CCAM)
- No peristalsis
- Diaphragm intact
- Abdominal circumference normal

Other Cystic Masses
- Bronchogenic cyst, neurenteric cyst, esophageal duplication cyst
- All rare
- More often associated with mediastinum

Pathology

General
- Associated abnormalities are common

Congenital Diaphragmatic Hernia

- o Structural
  - Central nervous system (CNS) malformations: 30%
  - Cardiac: 20%
  - Renal
  - Spinal
- o Chromosomal
  - Trisomy 18
  - Trisomy 21
  - All fetuses should be karyotyped
- o Multiple syndromes including Fryns and Beckwith-Wiedemann
- Genetics
  - o Generally sporadic inheritance
- Embryology
  - o Failure of fusion of the posterior pleuroperitoneal membranes
- Epidemiology
  - o 1:2,000 to 1:3,000 births

Clinical Issues
Clinical Presentation
- May be an incidental finding
- Patient may be large-for-dates secondary to polyhydramnios
Treatment
- In utero repair not shown to be useful
- Tracheal occlusion appears promising
  - o Causes retention of fetal lung fluid which accelerates lung growth
  - o Performed before 26 weeks gestational age on fetuses with poor prognosis
    - "Liver-up"
    - LHR < 1.0
  - o Necessitates delivery by cesarean section using **EXIT procedure** (ex utero intrapartum treatment)
    - Placental circulation is maintained while tracheal clip is removed and fetus intubated
- Majority repaired after delivery
- Severe cases may require extracorporeal membrane oxygenation (ECMO)
Prognosis
- Two major factors
  - o Presence of other abnormalities
  - o Degree of pulmonary hypoplasia
- Other poor prognostic factors
  - o Diagnosis before 24 weeks gestational age
  - o Large size
  - o **Liver in chest**
    - Mortality "liver-up" 57%
    - Mortality "liver-down" 7%

Selected References
1. Leung JWT et al: Prenatal MR imaging of congenital diaphragmatic hernia. AJR 174:1607-12, 2000
2. Lipshutz GS et al: Prospective analysis of lung-to-head ratio predicts survival for patients with prenatally diagnosed congenital diaphragmatic hernia. J Pediatr Surg 32:1634-6, 1997
3. Adzick NS et al: Diaphragmatic hernia in the fetus: Prenatal diagnosis and outcome in 94 cases. J Pediatr Surg 20:357-61, 1985

Pleural Effusion

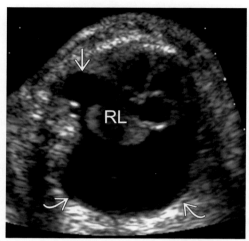

Pleural effusion. A right-sided chylothorax (curved arrows) displaces the heart and mediastinum into the left chest. Note that some of the fluid has herniated into the left chest as well (straight arrow). The right lung (RL) is markedly compressed by fluid.

Key Facts
- Synonyms: Hydrothorax, chylothorax, pleural fluid
- Definition: Accumulation of fluid in pleural space
- Classic imaging appearance: Curvilinear collection of fluid that displaces lung away from chest wall and diaphragm
- Can be from a primary congenital defect of lymphatics (chylothorax) or secondary to a systemic problem (hydrothorax)
- **Chylothorax** usually **unilateral**; rarely with hydrops fetalis
- **Hydrothorax** usually **bilateral**; often with **hydrops fetalis**
- In utero treatment possible with thoracentesis

Imaging Findings
General Features
- Best imaging clue: As anechoic pleural fluid accumulates, **lung appears to "float"** in chest
Ultrasound Findings
- Routine transverse view at level of four-chamber heart shows curvilinear anechoic fluid displacing lung away from chest wall and diaphragm
- Coronal views show "wing-like" lungs "floating" in chest
- **Any amount of pleural fluid is abnormal**
- Will appear anechoic regardless of chylothorax or hydrothorax
- Chylothorax appearance
  - **Unilateral** pleural effusion: Right = left
  - Often see mass effect
    - Mediastinal shift
    - Flattened diaphragm
  - Associated with trisomy 21 and Turner syndrome (2-6% risk)
    - If < 15 weeks, then association is very strong
- Hydrothorax
  - **Bilateral and symmetric** without mass effect

Pleural Effusion

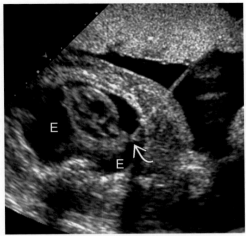

Bilateral pleural effusions. Therapeutic thoracentesis is performed in this fetus with bilateral pleural effusions (E) and hydrops fetalis (note the skin thickening). A needle is guided into the pleural space (needle tip - curved arrow) and fluid is removed prior to delivery.

- o Associated with immune and non-immune **hydrops fetalis**
  - ▪ Ascites, skin edema, pleural fluid, pericardial fluid
  - ▪ Look for anomalies and other causes of hydrops
- Pleural effusion rarely seen with chest masses
  - o Extralobar pulmonary sequestration
    - ▪ 5-10% develop tension hydrothorax
  - o Pulmonary lymphangiectasia
  - o Cystic adenomatoid malformation

Imaging Recommendations
- Try to distinguish between primary and secondary causes
- Look for other anomalies (30%)
- Sequential ultrasound to look for hydrops or increasing fluid
- Consider thoracentesis for treatment

Differential Diagnosis
Normal Chest Wall Musculature
- Chest wall muscles and diaphragm are hypoechoic (not anechoic) and should not be confused with pleural effusion

Pathology
General
- Genetics
  - o Associated with **Trisomy 21, Turner and Noonan** syndromes
  - o Congenital lymphatic disorders may present with pleural effusion
- Etiology-Pathogenesis
  - o Embryology: Chylothorax
    - ▪ Atresia, fistula or absence of **thoracic duct**
    - ▪ Thoracic duct crosses from right to left at 5th thoracic level
    - ▪ Equally right and left sided depending on level of obstruction

Pleural Effusion

- o Etiology
  - Hydrothorax from any cause of hydrops fetalis (immune and nonimmune)
  - 30% with nonimmune hydrops have anomalies (often cardiac)
- Epidemiology
  - o 1:15,000 pregnancies

Clinical Issues

Presentation
- Abnormal screening exam or in association with hydrops fetalis

Natural History
- Spontaneous resolution of primary chylothorax in 15%
- Unilateral effusion may rarely lead to hydrops fetalis
- Bilateral effusions may be earliest sign of impending hydrops fetalis
- Increased risk for pulmonary hypoplasia when untreated

Treatment
- Reasons to treat
  - o **Pulmonary hypoplasia**
  - o Immediately before delivery to aid with postnatal ventilation
- No treatment necessary if unilateral, small, and well tolerated
- If associated with hydrops fetalis, treat cause of hydrops
- If large or increasing with time, treat for impending pulmonary hypoplasia
- **Fetal thoracentesis** with ultrasound guidance
  - o Initial aspiration performed
  - o Fluid sent to lab to determine chylothorax vs hydrothorax
    - Chylothorax has high levels of lipoprotein and lymphocytes
  - o Chlothorax fluid is clear (not milky) since fetus is "fasting"
- **Thoracoamniotic shunting**
  - o Reaccumulated fluid after fetal thoracentesis
  - o Allows for continuous drainage
  - o Double pigtail catheter placed via trocar
    - Internal loop in chest and external loop in amniotic fluid
  - o 30% shunt failure rate

Prognosis
- Variable depending on size and presence of hydrops
- 35-50% mortality rates for all cases
- 2-6% risk for chromosome aneuploidy with chylothorax

Selected References
1. Aubard Y et al: Primary fetal hydrothorax: a literature review and proposed antenatal clinical strategy. Fetal Diagn Ther 1998:325-33, 1998
2. Hagay Z et al: Isolated fetal pleural effusion: A prenatal management dilemma. Obstet Gynecol 81:147-52, 1993
3. Petrikovsky BM et al: Pleural effusion in aneuploidy. Am J Perinatol 8:214-6, 1991

PocketRadiologist®

Obstetrics
Top 100 Diagnoses

CARDIAC

Normal Heart

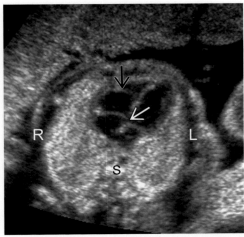

Normal heart, 4-chamber view. Fetal spine (S) is posterior and apex points to left. Atria and ventricles are symmetric. The tricuspid valve insertion (white arrow) is more apical than the mitral. Moderator band (black arrow) confirms that right ventricle is anterior.

Key Facts
- Definition: Normal configuration of atria, ventricles, valves, and outflow tracts
- Classic imaging appearance: **Normal 4-chamber (4-C) view excludes up to 90% congenital heart disease (CHD)**
- **Outflow tracts essential part of cardiac exam**
- Conotruncal malformations almost always normal on 4-C
  - Clinically relevant lesions for neonate are easily missed
    - Tetralogy of Fallot (ToF)
    - Truncus Arteriosus (TA)
    - Transposition of Great Vessels (TGV)
- Other significant CHD with normal 4-chamber view
  - Total anomalous pulmonary venous return (TAPVR)
  - Partial anomalous pulmonary venous return (PAPVR)

Imaging Findings
<u>General Features</u>
- Best imaging clue: Normal 4-C **and** outflow tract views
- Position
  - Apex left
  - Axis approximately 45 degrees off midline
    - Measure axis between plane of septum and line from spine to anterior chest (goes through LA, RV)
- Size
  - Atria/ventricles symmetric
  - Length atrial septum: Ventricular septum = 1:2
  - Heart occupies 1/3rd area of chest in 4-C view
  - Cardiac circumference about half chest circumference
- Rate and rhythm
  - Sinus rhythm

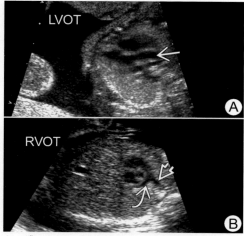

Normal heart, outflow tracts. (A) LVOT (white arrow) exits left ventricle & runs to right of midline before forming aortic arch. (B) RVOT curves around the aortic root, which is central in the heart. It branches into ductus (open arrow), which runs posteriorly toward the spine and the right pulmonary artery (curved arrow).

- o 120-160 beats per minute
- o Observe for 30 seconds
- o Record rhythm with M-mode or Doppler
- Contractility
  - o Assess ventricular function real time
  - o Ventricular "squeeze" should be equal

Ultrasound Findings

- **4-chamber view**
  - o Ventricles approximately equal in diameter
    - Measure at level of AV valves
    - Changes as pregnancy progresses
    - RV:LV = 1:1 at 18 weeks
    - RV:LV = 1.6:1 at term
  - o Apex of both ventricles at same level
  - o Interventricular septum intact
  - o Interatrial septum intact except for foramen ovale
    - Flap opens from RA to LA
  - o **Tricuspid valve inserted more toward apex** than mitral
    - Offset may increase from 2-9 mm from 20 weeks to term
- Chamber identification
  - o Right atrium receives hepatic veins
  - o **Right ventricle has moderator band**
  - o Left atrium receives pulmonary veins
  - o Left ventricle has 2 papillary muscles
- AV valves "belong" to ventricle
  - o Mitral to LV/tricuspid to RV
- **Outflow tracts**: Cross as they exit heart
  - o Right ventricular outflow tract (RVOT)
    - Anterior to left ventricular outflow tract (LVOT)

Normal Heart

- Runs right to left
- "Bifurcates" early ⇒ ductus arteriosus (DA), right pulmonary (RPA)
- Anatomical trifurcation ⇒ DA, RPA, left pulmonary artery (LPA)
- Only two branches seen in this scan plane
  - o Left ventricular (LVOT)
    - Posterior to RVOT, central in heart
    - Runs left to right
- "Arches"
  - o **Aortic**
    - Higher, curved arch: **"Candy cane"**
    - Gives rise to neck vessels
  - o **Ductal**
    - Shorter, flatter arch: **"Hockey stick"**
    - Ductus arteriosus ⇒ runs toward spine to join descending aorta

Imaging Recommendations
- Aim to image outflow tracts in all patients
- Evaluate cardiac structure in **step-wise fashion**
  - o Veins ⇒ atria
  - o Atria ⇒ ventricles
  - o Ventricles ⇒ outflow portion
  - o Outflow portion ⇒ great vessels

Differential Diagnosis
Conotruncal Malformations
- **Poor prenatal detection if outflow tracts not evaluated**
Ventricular Septal Defect
- 30% missed on 4-C view
Atrial Septal Defect
- Rarely detected unless large
- Normal "defect" (foramen ovale)

Pathology
General
- Embryology
  - o Critical period days 20-50 post fertilization
  - o Initial tubular structure with sacculations
  - o Sinus venosus ⇒ trium ⇒ entricle ⇒ bulbus cordis ⇒ truncus arteriosus
  - o Tube loops and partitions to form four chambers by end fourth week
  - o Pharyngeal arches ⇒ aortic arches 4th to 5th weeks
  - o Adult arrangement of arches between 6th and 8th weeks

Clinical Issues
Presentation
- Adequate views in majority of patients by 14 weeks
Prognosis
- Excellent

Selected References
1. Huggon IC et al: Fetal cardiac abnormalities identified prior to 14 weeks gestation. Ultrasound Obstet Gynecol 20:22-9, 2002
2. Bull C et al: Current and potential impact of fetal diagnosis on prevalence and spectrum of serious congenital heart disease at term in the UK. Lancet 354:1242-7, 1999
3. Allan D et al: Anatomical and echocardiographic correlates of normal cardiac morphology in the late first trimester fetus. Heart 77:68-72, 1997

Hypoplastic Left Heart

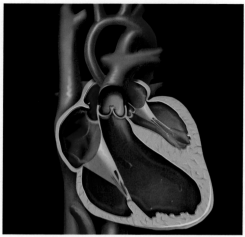

Hypoplastic left heart. Drawing depicts asymmetry of ventricular size and hypoplasia of aorta. Arch often fills retrograde via ductus, leading to ductal dependence. Apex of the left ventricle is proximal to right.

Key Facts
- Synonyms: Hypoplastic left heart syndrome (HLHS), hypoplastic left ventricle (LV), aortic atresia
- Definition: Atresia or hypoplasia LV
- Classic imaging appearance: Small or absent LV
- Often associated atresia/hypoplasia of
  - Ascending aorta
  - Aortic valve
  - Mitral valve

Imaging Findings
<u>General Features</u>
- Best imaging clue: Inability to show symmetric ventricles on 4-chamber view
<u>Ultrasound Findings</u>
- Left ventricle
  - Small or invisible
  - May be globular
  - Hypocontractile
  - Echogenic wall
  - Apex LV proximal to apex right ventricle (RV)
- Right ventricle
  - Looks large
  - Apex RV distal to apex LV
- Atria
  - Left < right
  - Inter-atrial septum bowed left to right
- Retrograde filling of arch and descending aorta
  - Transverse view superior mediastinum: Transverse arch, ductus
  - Color Doppler: Reverse arch flow = ductal dependence

Hypoplastic Left Heart

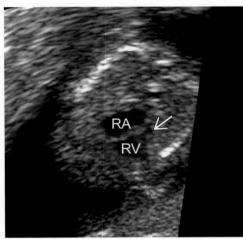

Hypoplastic left heart. Ultrasound image at level of four-chamber view is well positioned (ribs are symmetric "C" shape). LV (arrow) is extremely small and was not contracting in real time. Right atrium (RA). Right ventricle (RV).

Imaging Recommendations
- Formal fetal echocardiogram looking for
  o Mitral stenosis/atresia
  o Aortic stenosis/atresia
  o Aortic arch interruption
  o Coarctation of the aorta: 80%
  o Endomyocardial fibroelastosis
  o Ventricular septal defect
- Full fetal survey: Central nervous system anomalies associated

Differential Diagnosis
Single Ventricle
- Aorta and pulmonary artery symmetric, arise from single ventricle
Severe Aortic Stenosis (AS)
- Antegrade flow across aortic valve
  o In HLH flow across aortic valve is absent or retrograde

Pathology
General
- Endomyocardial fibroelastosis (EFE) may progress to HLHS
- Genetics
  o Transcription factor gene mutations: Not hereditary
- Embryology
  o Abnormal partitioning of primitive conotruncus into left and right ventricular outflow tracts
  o Hypoplasia/atresia of aortic valve
  o Diminished antegrade flow through aorta
    ▪ Underdevelopment of left ventricle and aorta "form follows function"

Hypoplastic Left Heart

- Epidemiology
  - 1-3:10,000 live births
  - 9% CHD
  - M:F = 2:1

Clinical Issues

Presentation

- Most cases detected on routine 18 to 20 week scan
- EFE/severe AS may $\Rightarrow$ HLH: May not be visible until third trimester
- 95% prenatal diagnoses confirmed

Natural History

- Most severe congenital heart lesion presenting in neonate
- Lethal in days/weeks if untreated

Treatment

- Offer karyotype: Chromosomal abnormality in 2-10%
- Offer termination
- Prenatal intervention: Experimental balloon valvuloplasty
  - Preliminary results poor
  - Selection criteria not established
- If pregnancy continued, family choose comfort care **or** surgical intervention
- Surgical intervention: Deliver at tertiary center
- Norwood three-stage procedure
  - Construction neo-aorta from pulmonary artery, atrial septectomy, Blalock-Taussig shunt for pulmonary perfusion (3 weeks)
  - Conversion to hemi-Fontan: Glenn shunt superior vena cava to right pulmonary artery (4–6 months)
  - Fontan: Fenestrated venous conduit through right atrium: Inferior vena cava flow to right pulmonary artery
- Neonatal cardiac transplant

Prognosis

- Prenatal diagnosis
  - 45% termination
  - 20% intrauterine fetal demise
  - 75% of those born alive die within first week
- Norwood
  - Stage 1 mortality rate 23-46%
  - Stage 2 mortality rate 3%
  - Stage 3 mortality rate 8%
- Heart transplant
  - 19% mortality on transplant list
  - 9% operative mortality
- Prenatal diagnosis = better perinatal stabilization
- Improving surgical techniques = increased survival
- Future prognosis may change significantly

Selected References
1. Meyer-Wittkopf M: Interventional fetal cardiac therapy-possible perspectives and current shortcomings. Ultrasound Obstet Gynecol 20:527-31, 2002
2. Vinals F et al: Prenatal diagnosis of ductal dependent congenital heart disease: How can things be made easier? Ultrasound Obstet Gynecol 19:246-9, 2002
3. Norwood WI: Hypoplastic left heart syndrome. Ann Thorac Surg 52:688-95, 1991

Ventricular Septal Defect

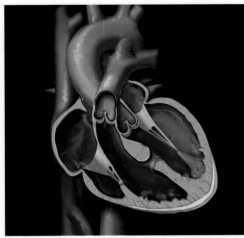

Ventricular septal defect (VSD). Drawing depicts muscular VSD. In the fetus right and left heart pressures are symmetric and the shunt is bi-directional, R $\Rightarrow$ L in systole, L $\Rightarrow$ R in late diastole.

Key Facts
- Definition: Defect in ventricular septum
- Classic imaging appearance: Area of signal dropout in ventricular septum
- Normal transition muscular to membranous septum mimics ventricular septal defect (VSD) on apical 4-chamber view
- Commonest congenital heart defect in children (not fetuses)
  - More complex heart defects seen in the fetus
- VSD > 50% aortic root $\Rightarrow$ functional significance in infancy
- Prenatal diagnosis of isolated VSD poor prognosis **but** isolated VSD has relatively good prognosis

Imaging Findings
General Features
- Best imaging clue: Aortic septal continuity best seen on left ventricle **long axis view**
  - Posterior wall aorta lined up with anterior cusp mitral valve
  - Septum should be continuous with anterior wall
  - Loss of continuity $\Rightarrow$ overriding aorta
- Membranous 80%
- Muscular 20%
  - Inlet
  - Trabecular
    - Small defects open in diastole
    - Narrow in systole
  - Outlet/infundibular/malalignment
    - Tetralogy of Fallot
    - Truncus arteriosus
    - Pulmonary atresia

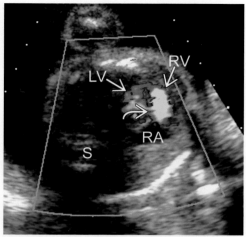

Ventricular septal defect. Color Doppler ultrasound confirms flow across membranous VSD (curved arrow). (RA - right atrium, RV - right ventricle, LV - left ventricle, S - spine).

Ultrasound Findings
- Signal drop out in septum
  - Echogenic reflector from edge of defect
  - Confirm on long axis view if seen on apical 4-chamber view
  - True VSD: Visible in **two scan planes**
- **Color Doppler** confirms blood flow across defect
  - RV/LV pressures similar in fetus
  - **Shunt bi-directional**
    - Systole R ⇒ L
    - Late diastole L ⇒ R
  - Unidirechonal shunt: Look for other anomalies
Imaging Recommendations
- Formal fetal echocardiography
  - 50% association with additional cardiac anomaly
- Complete structural survey

Differential Diagnosis
Complete Atrioventricular Septal Defect
- Defect involves atrial and ventricular septa
- Single valve in center of heart
Partial Atrioventricular Septal Defect
- Defect involves inferior atrial septum not ventricular septum

Pathology
General
- Genetics
  - Holt-Oram Syndrome: Autosomal dominant
    - Atrial/ventricular septal defects
    - Radial ray and other skeletal malformations
    - Mutation of gene encoding TBX5 transcription factor

Ventricular Septal Defect

- Etiology-Pathogenesis
  - Teratogen exposure
    - Lithium
    - Isotretinoin
    - Phenytoin
    - Oral contraceptives
- Epidemiology
  - 1:5,000 total births
  - 30% congenital heart disease (CHD) in liveborn
  - 10% fetal CHD
  - Disparity due to demise of fetuses with more complex CHD
  - M > F

Clinical Issues
Presentation
- **30% missed on 4-chamber view**
- Consider first trimester EV scans in high-risk patient
  - Satisfactory views in 92% at 13 weeks
Treatment
- Karyotype: Reported aneuploidy association 18-70%
- Prenatal pediatric cardiology consultation
- Large VSD ⇒ risk early decompensation ⇒ consider delivery at tertiary center
- Monitor growth
- Follow for development of hydrops
  - Low risk with isolated small VSD
Prognosis
- Variable, depends on
  - Size of defect
  - Degree left-right shunt
  - Associated cardiac abnormalities: Occur in 50%
- Up to 74% spontaneous closure in utero
- Liveborn, isolated VSD
  - 40% spontaneous closure by age 1
  - 50% by age 5
  - 80% by adolescence
- Surgical repair if maximal medical therapy fails
  - Right atrial approach, Dacron patch, cardiopulmonary bypass
  - Operative mortality < 5%
- Recurrence risk
  - One child 3%
  - Two children 10%
  - Maternal VSD: 6-10%
  - Paternal VSD: 2%

Selected References
1. Haak MC et al: How successful is fetal echocardiographic examination in the first trimester of pregnancy? Ultrasound Obstet Gynecol 20:9-13, 2002
2. Paladini D et al: Characterization and natural history of ventricular septal defects in the fetus. Ultrasound Obstet Gynecol 16:118-22, 2000
3. Chao RC et al: Fluctuations of interventricular shunting in a fetus with isolated VSD. Am Heart J 127:955-8, 1994

Atrioventricular Septal Defect

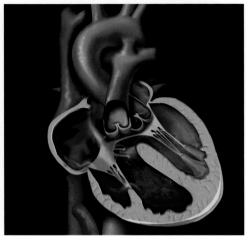

Atrioventricular septal defect. Drawing depicts aorta and pulmonary artery straddling central defect in the heart. Great vessels and chambers are equal in size in the fetus. The usual offset of mitral and tricuspid valves on the interventricular septum is absent due to the presence of a central common valve.

Key Facts
- Synonyms: Endocardial cushion defect, atrioventricular (AV) canal
- Definition: Central defect in heart involving atrial and ventricular septa, atrioventricular valves +/- conducting system
- Classic imaging appearance: Central defect on 4-chamber view
- Anatomy: Complete or partial
  - Complete: ASD, VSD, common AV valve
  - Partial: Ostium primum ASD, common AV valve
- Atrioventricular septal defect (AVSD) as isolated cardiac defect ⇒ **Down syndrome > 50%**
- AVSD + additional cardiac anomaly ⇒ heterotaxia syndromes

Imaging Findings
General Features
- Best imaging clue: **Missing "crux" of the heart in diastole** on 4-chamber view
Ultrasound Findings
- Single **AV valve makes straight line** across heart in **systole**
  - Tricuspid normally 1-2 mm offset from mitral insertion ⇒ "crux"
- Associated with bradycardia: Conduction system involved in defect
- Heterotaxia syndromes
  - Right atrial isomerism 50%
    - Bilateral "right-sided" bronchi
    - Asplenia
    - Pulmonary stenosis +/- double outlet right ventricle
    - Anomalous pulmonary venous drainage
  - Left atrial isomerism 20%
    - Bilateral "left-sided" bronchi
    - Polysplenia

Atrioventricular Septal Defect

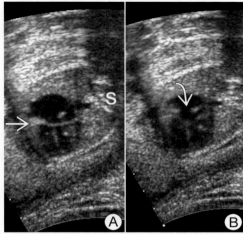

Atrioventricular septal defect. Ultrasound four-chamber view in systole (A) and diastole (B). The common AV valve forms a single echo (arrow) when closed. In diastole the valve opens centrally in the heart (curved arrow). VSD is better seen in diastole. Anhydramnios secondary to co-existent renal agenesis. (S – spine).

- Azygos continuation inferior vena cava
- Complete heart block

Imaging Recommendations
- Formal fetal echocardiogram
  - 70% additional cardiac anomaly
    - Tetralogy of Fallot
    - Aortic coarctation
    - Pulmonary stenosis
    - Double outlet right ventricle
    - Atrial isomerism
  - Pansystolic AV valve regurgitation: High incidence of hydrops
  - Early systolic AV valve regurgitation: Better prognosis
  - Ventricular dominance: Impacts surgical outcome
- Partial form may have only small defect in inferior atrial septum: Prenatal diagnosis harder
- Full survey for other anomalies
  - 76% children (not fetuses) have a syndrome

Differential Diagnosis
Large VSD
- AV valves normal
Large ASD
- AV valves normal

Pathology
General
- Genetics
  - Associated with trisomy 21, 8p- deletion 50%
  - Can be syndromic

Atrioventricular Septal Defect

- Embryology
  - Endocardial cushions fail to fuse
  - Primitive AV canal persists after 6 weeks gestational age
- Epidemiology
  - 0.11-0.36/1,000 live births
  - 1-5% CHD
  - Fetal incidence = 4x liveborn
  - Fetal complete AVSD = 97%
  - Postnatal complete AVSD = 69%

Clinical Issues
Presentation
- Complete AV canal detected as early as 12 to 14 weeks with endovaginal scanning

Treatment
- Encourage amniocentesis: 50% association with chromosome abnormality
- Offer termination
- If pregnancy continues, refer to tertiary center for delivery
- Prenatal consultation with pediatric cardiologist and neonatologist
- Not indication for early delivery or C-section
  - Low birth weight increases risk from cardiac surgery

Prognosis
- Extremely poor if
  - Multiple congenital anomalies
  - Hydrops
  - Left atrial isomerism: 85% fetal demise
  - Right atrial isomerism: High infant mortality
- Trisomy 21 not **independent** risk factor for adverse surgical outcome
  - Trisomy 21 infants have same surgical outcome as those with normal chromosomes
- Untreated
  - 50% mortality in first six months
  - 80% mortality in first year
- Surgical repair
  - 5% operative mortality
  - 90% survivors have normal function
  - 85% 12-year survival rate
- Recurrence risk
  - One child: 3%
  - Two children: 10%
  - Parent with AV canal and normal chromosomes: 10%
    - Higher for affected mother than father

Selected References
1. Pierpont M et al: Genetic aspects of atrioventricular septal defects. Am J Med Genet 97:289-96, 2000
2. Allen LD et al: Atrioventricular septal defects in the fetus. Am J Obstet Gynecol 181:1250-3, 1999
3. Achiron R et al: First trimester diagnosis of fetal congenital heart diseases by transvaginal ultrasonography. Obstet Gynecol 84:69-72, 1994

Tetralogy of Fallot

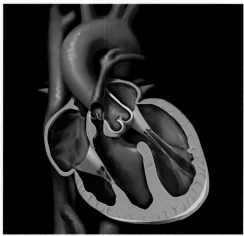

Tetralogy of fallot. Drawing depicts pulmonary infundibular stenosis. Right and left heart pressures are equal in the fetus therefore ventricles are symmetric. Aorta appears large due to relative decrease in blood flow through pulmonary artery. Aortic root overrides ventricular septal defect (VSD).

Key Facts
- Definition: Composed of four components
  - Ventricular septal defect (VSD)
  - Overriding aorta
  - Right ventricular hypertrophy
  - Right ventricular outflow tract (RVOT) obstruction
    - **Infundibular stenosis 100%**
    - Valve stenosis +/-
    - **Pulmonary atresia ⇒ dismal prognosis**
    - Absent pulmonary valve ⇒ enlarged pulmonary artery (PA)
- Right and left heart pressures almost **equal** in fetus
- RVOT obstruction not hemodynamically significant in the fetus
  - 11% of fetal cardiac output to lungs

Imaging Findings
General Features
- Best imaging clue: Dilated aortic root overriding VSD
Ultrasound Findings
- **4 chamber view normal in > 95%** prenatal cases
- **Outflow tract assessment key**
- 3-vessel view abnormal in majority
  - Transverse view upper mediastinum
  - Normal: Main PA, ascending aorta, superior vena cava
  - Tetralogy: PA small, aorta displaced anteriorly
- Aortic outflow large, root overrides high VSD
- Ductus arteriosus small in 70%, not visualized in rest
- Absent pulmonary valve complex (APVC): Increased risk of hydrops
  - APVC + hydrops = 80% mortality
- Doppler: Turbulent flow across RVOT

Tetralogy of Fallot

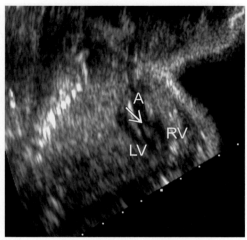

Tetralogy of fallot. Sagittal image through the heart shows a large anteriorly displaced aorta (A) overriding a high VSD (arrow). Right (RV) and left (LV) ventricles are equal in size in the fetus as RVOT obstruction not hemodynamically significant.

<u>Imaging Recommendations</u>
- Formal fetal echocardiogram for
  - APVC/pulmonary atresia ⇒ worse prognosis
- Detailed anatomic survey
  - Increased risk of aneuploidy if other anomalies
- Follow for development of hydrops
  - 17-41% mortality

Differential Diagnosis
<u>Truncus Arteriosus</u>
- Single vessel leaves heart
  - 65% arise primarily from RV
  - 15% only from RV
  - **Only 15% straddle VSD**
- Pulmonary arteries arise from truncal vessel
- Truncal valve has 2-5 leaflets
<u>Double Outlet Right Ventricle (DORV)</u>
- Great vessels parallel as exit heart
- More than 90% surface area of great vessel roots must arise from RV
- Technically Fallot with majority of aortic root to right of VSD = DORV
<u>Pulmonary Atresia With VSD</u>
- Abnormal 4-chamber view: Small RV, large RA
- No antegrade flow across pulmonary valve
- Retrograde flow in ductus arteriosus

Pathology
<u>General</u>
- Genetics
  - Trisomy 13, 18

Tetralogy of Fallot

- o 22q11 deletion
- Embryology
  - o Abnormal conotruncal septation
  - o Abnormal bulbotruncal rotation
  - o Primary hypoplasia of infundibular septum
- Syndromic association
  - o CHARGE
    - Coloboma
    - Heart disease
    - Atresia (choanal)
    - Restricted growth/development
    - Genital anomalies
    - Ear/hearing defects
  - o VACTERL association
  - o Velocardiofacial/Di George syndrome
- Epidemiology
  - o 3-5:10,000 live births
  - o 5-10% of CHD in live born
  - o Fourth most common congenital heart anomaly

Clinical Issues

Presentation
- As early as 14 weeks on endovaginal US

Treatment
- Encourage karyotype
  - o Abnormal in 50% prenatal cases
  - o Abnormal in 12% live born
- Prenatal consultation with pediatric cardiologist
- Deliver at tertiary center
- Consider delivery at lung maturity if hydropic
- Prenatal diagnosis
  - o 18-41% termination of pregnancy
  - o 27-55% neonatal death
  - o 27-32% survival
- Surgical repair
  - o 93-98% survival for repair of Tetralogy with pulmonary stenosis if normal chromosomes and no other anomaly
- Recurrence risk
  - o One child 2.5%
  - o Two children 8%
  - o Mother 2.5%
  - o Father 1.5%

Selected References
1. Moon-Grady AJ et al: Value of clinical and echocardiographic features in predicting outcome in the fetus, infant and child with Tetralogy of Fallot and absent pulmonary valve complex. Am J Card 89:1280-5, 2002
2. Yoo SJ et al: Tetralogy of Fallot in the fetus: Findings at targeted sonography. Ultrasound Obstet Gynecol 14:29-37, 1999
3. Achiron R et al: Transvaginal echocardiographic examination of the fetal heart between 13 and 15 weeks gestation in a low risk population. J Ultrasound Med 13:783-9, 1994

Pericardial Effusion

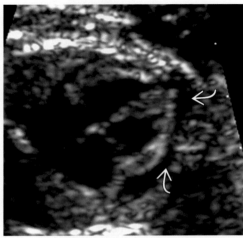

Pericardial effusion. A small amount of fluid is seen adjacent to the fetal heart (curved arrows). The fluid measured 3 mm, and follow-up examination was performed. The pericardial effusion worsened, heart size increased, and the fetus developed hydrops fetalis secondary to cardiomyopathy.

Key Facts
- Synonym: Pericardial fluid
- Definition: Accumulation of **fluid in pericardial space**
- Classic imaging appearance: Pericardial effusion (PE) completely or partially surrounds fetal heart
- **Small amount of fluid (< 2 mm) considered normal**
- May be transient
- May be early sign of **hydrops fetalis**
- Associated with **cardiac anomalies and arrhythmia**

Imaging Findings
General Features
- Best imaging clue: Fluid collection, measuring > 2 mm, surrounds fetal heart
- When large, heart is seen beating in a "bag of water"

Ultrasound Findings
- Lenticular or oval collection of fluid adjacent to, or surrounding heart
- **Seen best on standard four-chamber view**
- May see normal trace fluid along one ventricular wall
  - Up to 2 mm of fluid considered normal
  - Majority of fetuses (50-80%) have trace of fluid if careful search done
  - If fetus not at increased risk, follow-up not necessary
- Associated with **hydrops fetalis**
  - **When PE seen early,** hydrops more likely associated with **cardiac abnormality**
    - Cardiac arrhythmia
    - Structural defect
    - Cardiomyopathy

Pericardial Effusion

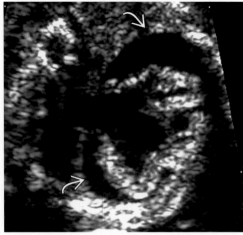

Pericardial effusion. A large amount of fluid surrounds this abnormal heart (curved arrows). The fetus had a complex cardiac anomaly and developed hydrops fetalis. The heart appears to be suspended in a "bag of fluid."

- o When PE seen late, hydrops likely from other causes
    - Infection
    - Noncardiac anomalies
    - Immune causes

Imaging Recommendations
- **Look for early signs of hydrops**
    - o Skin edema
    - o Pleural effusion
    - o Ascites
- Look for signs of **congenital infection**
    - o Liver and brain calcifications
    - o Echogenic bowel
- Cardiac anomalies
- M-mode evaluation of fetal heart for **arrhythmia**
- Perform formal fetal echocardiography
- Follow-up exams necessary when fluid is > 2 mm or in high risk patients
    - o Progression to hydrops
    - o Complete resolution of PE

Differential Diagnosis
Normal Pericardial Fluid
- Less than 2 mm
- May be transient
- Follow-up ultrasound in high risk patients

Normal Peripheral Myocardium
- Outside 1-6 mm of myocardium may be hypoechoic and mimic fluid
- Circular outer muscle fibers cause this effect
- Look for contracting rim
    - o Contracting heart and immobile ring with PE

Pleural Effusion
- Usually not just adjacent to heart
  - Look along ribs
- Rarely asymmetric and mimics pericardial effusion

Pathology
General
- Etiology-Pathogenesis
  - Cardiac abnormality
    - Arrhythmia, anatomic defect, cardiomyopathy
    - PE may be the first sign of hydrops
  - Immune hydrops fetalis
    - Ascites usually the first sign
    - PE when hydrops is severe
  - Congenital infection
    - CMV, toxoplasmosis, rubella, Parvovirus B19, syphilis

Clinical Issues
Presentation
- Abnormal screening exam
- In association with hydrops fetalis
- In association with cardiac anomaly
Treatment
- No treatment necessary if isolated and small
- Underlying cause treated
- Pharmaceutical treatment for arrhythmias
  - Digoxin, flecainide, amiodarone, procainamide, adenosine
Prognosis
- Variable depending on cause

Selected References
1.   Yoo SJ et al: Normal pericardial fluid in the fetus: Color and spectral Doppler analysis. Ultrasound Obstet Gynecol 18:248-52, 2001
2.   Dizon-Townson DS et al: A prospective evaluation of fetal pericardial fluid in 506 second trimester low-risk pregnancies. Obstet Gynecol 90:958-61, 1997
3.   Shenker L et al: Fetal pericardial effusion. Am J Obstet Gynecol 160:1505-8, 1989

Rhabdomyoma

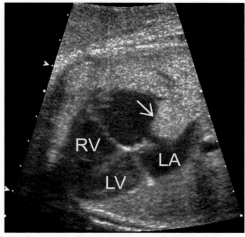

Right atrial rhabdomyoma. Four-chamber view of the heart shows an echogenic mass involving the upper portion of the atrial septum (arrow). (LV - left ventricle, RV - right ventricle, LA - left atrium).

Key Facts
- Definition: Congenital cardiac hamartoma composed of abnormal myocytes
- Classic imaging appearance: Echogenic intracardiac mass
- Most common in utero finding of **tuberous sclerosis** (TS)
  - 50-85% of fetuses with rhabdomyomas have TS
  - 50% of fetuses with TS have rhabdomyomas
- May be multiple in 50%
  - Increases likelihood of TS

Imaging Findings
General Features
- Best imaging clue: Well-defined, hyperechoic, intracardiac mass
Ultrasound Findings
- Small masses within wall may appear as wall thickening
- Other findings in tuberous sclerosis
  - Tubers
    - Often difficult to discern
    - Look for contour irregularities of ventricle
MR Findings
- Helpful to evaluate for CNS findings in TS
  - Tubers hyperintense on T1WI
Imaging Recommendations
- Look for findings of TS
- Cardiac echo
  - Evaluate for
    - Outflow obstruction
    - Valvular insufficiency
    - Arrhythmia
    - Hydrops

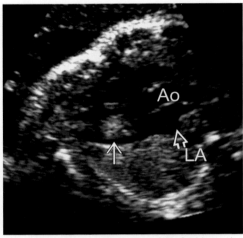

Left ventricular rhabdomyoma. Long-axis view of the fetal heart showing the left ventricular outflow tract demonstrates an echogenic mass within the left ventricle (arrow). (LA - left atrium, AO – ascending aorta).

- Minority have associated structural defect

Differential Diagnosis
<u>Other Cardiac Tumors (All Rare)</u>
- All are solitary masses
  - Rhabdomyomas are frequently multiple
- Teratoma
  - Pericardial (not myocardial) tumor
    - Exophytic growth (will not be in cardiac chamber)
  - Heterogeneous with calcification
- Hemangioma
- Fibroma
  - Ventricular apex
- Myxomas not seen in utero
<u>Echogenic Cardiac Focus</u>
- Papillary muscle
- Small
- Very bright (similar to bone)
<u>Hypertrophic Cardiomyopathy</u>
- Diffuse wall thickening
  - Left ventricle most common
- **Diabetic mothers** in 90%
  - Poor control
<u>Endocardial Fibroelastosis</u>
- Echogenic endocardium and papillary muscles
- Poor contractility

Pathology
<u>General</u>
- General Path Comments

Rhabdomyoma

- o Diagnosed after 20 weeks
- o Most commonly on ventricular septum but may be anywhere
- o Features of TS
  - Clinical triad: Seizures, mental retardation, cutaneous angiofibromas
  - Cardiac: Rhabdomyomas (**most common in utero finding**)
  - Brain: Cortical tubers, subependymal nodules (rarely seen in utero)
  - Renal: Angiomyolipomas and cysts (not seen in utero)
- Genetics
  - o TS autosomal dominant with > 50% new mutations

Gross Pathologic, Surgical Features
- Encapsulated intramyocardial or exophytic mass

Microscopic Features
- Large vacuolated myocytes
- Glycogen-rich vacuoles stretch the perinuclear cytoplasm (spider cells)

Clinical Issues

Presentation
- Generally incidental finding
- Rarely presents with arrhythmia or hydrops

Natural History
- Variable course
  - o Majority remain stable or even regress in utero
  - o May be complicated by arrhythmia, hydrops, and even death
  - o Most regress in infancy

Treatment
- Genetic counseling for TS
- Cardiac evaluation after delivery
- **Most regress without treatment**
  - o Both in TS and isolated abnormality
- Surgical resection if symptomatic

Prognosis
- Good if no complications in utero or first 6 months of life
- Cognitive function impaired in TS

Selected References
1. Axt-Fliedner R et al: Prenatal diagnosis of cerebral lesions and multiple intracardiac rhabdomyomas in a fetus with tuberous sclerosis. J Ultrasound Med 20:63-7, 2001
2. Holley DG et al: Diagnosis and management of fetal cardiac tumors: A multicenter experience and review of published reports. J Am Coll Cardiol 26:516-20, 1995
3. Groves AM et al: Cardiac tumours in intrauterine life. Arch Dis Child 67:1189-92, 1992

Arrhythmias

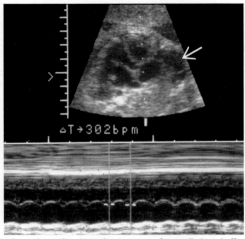

Supraventricular tachycardia. Note the presence of a small pleural effusion (arrow). The fetus converted to normal sinus rhythm with digoxin treatment.

Key Facts
- Definition: An abnormal heart rhythm manifested as
  - Tachycardia > 200 bpm
  - Bradycardia < 100 bpm
  - Irregular rhythm
- Classic imaging appearance: Abnormal Doppler tracing
- Premature atrial contractions **(PACs) account for 80% of cases**
  - Benign and self-limited
- Supraventricular tachycardia **(SVT) most common tachyarrhythmia**
  - Can lead to hydrops and death if untreated
- **Bradycardia** most often associated with **structural cardiac defects or maternal connective tissue diseases**

Imaging Findings
General Features
- Best imaging clue: Presence of an arrhythmia can usually be detected by careful observation
  - M-mode tracing must be performed to determine type
Ultrasound Findings
- Place M-mode cursor to include both atrium and ventricle
  - Evaluate atrial and ventricular rates and AV (atrioventricular) conduction
    - Is every atrial contraction followed by a ventricular contraction
- Transient sinus bradycardia may be caused by excessive transducer pressure
  - Vagal response
  - Heart rate will quickly return to normal when pressure is decreased
- Cardiac defects may be present especially if bradycardia
Imaging Recommendations
- Look for any evidence of hydrops including pericardial effusion

Arrhythmias

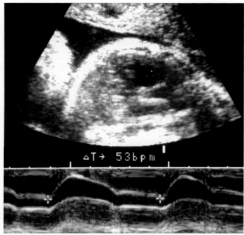

Severe sinus bradycardia in a fetus with an atrioventricular septal defect. There was in utero demise 2 days after the ultrasound exam.

- Dedicated fetal echo for significant arrhythmia (any other than PACs or premature ventricular contractions)
  - o Structural defects
  - o Valvular incompetence
  - o Hemodynamic decompensation

Differential Diagnosis
Premature Atrial Contraction
- 80% of arrhythmias
- Usually **transient and benign**
- Types
  - o Nonconducted: Early in cardiac cycle, no ventricular contraction
  - o Conducted: Later in cardiac cycle, results in ventricular contraction
- < 1% develop SVT
Premature Ventricular Contraction (PVC)
- Less common than PACs
- Also transient and benign
Tachycardia
- Rate > 200 bpm
- Types
  - o SVT most common
    - Atrial and ventricular rate the same
  - o Atrial flutter
    - Atrial rate is faster than ventricular rate (AV block, usually 2:1)
    - More likely to have structural defect than SVT
  - o Sinus tachycardia may be response to maternal condition
    - Thyrotoxicosis, fever, sepsis, or drugs
- **Can lead to cardiac compromise**, hydrops, and death
- Requires referral and treatment
  - o **Most fetuses will respond to therapy** but multiple drugs may be needed

Arrhythmias

Bradycardia
- Rate < 100 bpm
- Types
  - Sinus bradycardia: Atrial and ventricular rate the same
  - Complete AV block
    - Atrial rate normal with slow independent ventricular rate
- **50% will have structural defect**
  - Poor prognosis
- **50% in mothers with connective tissue diseases**
  - Maternal antibodies cross placenta and affect fetal conduction system
  - **Most survive despite complete AV block**
    - 10-15% mortality
  - Approximately 10% recurrence risk

Pathology
General
- Epidemiology
  - 2% of pregnancies will have arrhythmia
  - Most benign and self-limited (PACs, PVCs)

Clinical Issues
Presentation
- Abnormal heart rate or rhythm noted on physical exam
Treatment
- PACs and PVCs usually none but consider limiting caffeine intake and cessation of smoking
  - Monitor rate in clinic, repeat US if fails to resolve or SVT develops
- Tachycardia treated by interrupting AV re-entry circuit
  - **Digoxin** first-line drug
    - May be given orally to mother or via umbilical vein
    - Maternal serum levels must be monitored
    - Fetal levels approximately 80% of maternal levels
    - **Hydropic fetuses do not attain same levels** as non-hydropic and often require multiple drugs
  - Other drugs including flecainide, quinidine, procainamide, adenosine, and amiodarone have been used
    - Must be done under close supervision
- Limited treatment for bradycardia
  - Steroids and beta agonists have been given
  - Cardiac pacing not proven successful
Prognosis
- Excellent for PACs and PVCs
- Good for tachycardia
  - Arrhythmias can occur in neonatal period
  - Postnatal cardiac evaluation required for all
- **Bradycardia with structural abnormality generally lethal**

Selected References
1. Simpson JM et al: Fetal tachycardias: Management and outcome of 127 consecutive cases. Heart 79:576-81, 1998
2. Schmidt KG et al: Perinatal outcome of fetal complete atrioventricular block: A multicenter experience. J Am Coll Cardiol 17:1360-6, 1991
3. Silverman NH et al: Recognition of fetal arrhythmias by echocardiography. J Clin Ultrasound 13:255-63, 1985

Ebstein Anomaly

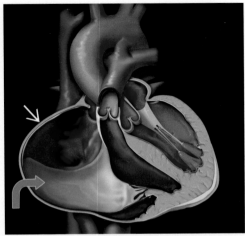

Ebstein anomaly. Drawing depicts large right atrium (arrow), non-contracting "atrialized" inlet portion of right ventricle (curved arrow) and small functional outlet portion of right ventricle.

Key Facts

- Definition
  - Apical displacement of septal and posterior tricuspid valve (TV) leaflets
  - Valve dysplasia + leaflet malposition = tricuspid regurgitation (TR)
  - Displaced leaflets adhere to wall inflow portion right ventricle (RV) ⇒ "atrialization" of right ventricle
- Lithium use is risk factor

Imaging Findings

General Features
- Best imaging clue: **Apical displacement of tricuspid valve**
  - Tricuspid normally lower on septum than mitral by 1-2 mm

Ultrasound Findings
- Apical displacement TV
- Large right atrium (RA) with atrialized portion of RV
- Small functional RV: Thin RV wall suggests RV dysplasia

Imaging Recommendations
- Formal fetal echocardiogram looking for
  - Rhythm: Associated with arrythmias
  - Tricuspid regurgitation
    - Severe TR ⇒ cardiomegaly ⇒ hydrops
  - Pulmonary stenosis
  - Associated structural abnormalities in 30%
    - Atrial/ventricular septal defect
    - Total anomalous pulmonary venous return
    - Mitral valve abnormalities
    - Coarctation of aorta
  - Cardiomegaly: Ratio heart circumference/chest circumference
    - Large heart ⇒ compressed lungs ⇒ pulmonary hypoplasia

Ebstein Anomaly

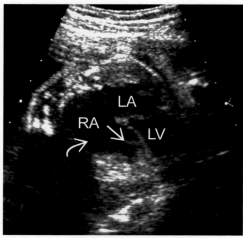

Ebstein anomaly. Four-chamber view shows massive cardiomegaly, with the heart occupying most of the thorax. Septal leaflet of tricuspid valve (arrow) is abnormally low on septum resulting in large RA/atrialized RV (curved arrow). Functional portion of RV is that part distal to septal leaflet insertion site.

▪ Left ventricle compressed by large right side structures

Differential Diagnosis
Tricuspid Regurgitation/Dysplasia
- TV incompetent **but normally located**
- Dysplastic valves thick, nodular, irregular
- Look for right heart obstruction as cause
  - Pulmonary atresia with intact ventricular septum
Pulmonary Atresia
- TV normally located
- Right atrium large
- RV may be hypoplastic but not atrialized
Uhl Anomaly
- TV normally located
- Hypoplasia RV myocardium

Pathology
General
- Etiology-Pathogenesis
  - First trimester maternal **lithium** exposure teratogenic
    - 400 x increased incidence compared to general population
    - 2.7% incidence in 225 exposed fetuses
    - First trimester lithium exposure: 2-3 x risk any congenital heart disease (CHD) in controlled studies
- Embryology
  - Inadequate separation TV leaflets and chordae tendineae from RV endocardium
- Epidemiology
  - 1/20,000 live births

- o 7% CHD in fetus
- o < 1% CHD in children
- o M = F

Clinical Issues
Presentation
- Detected on 4-chamber view at 18 weeks scan

Natural History
- Predisposes to arrythmias
  - o Supraventricular tachycardia
  - o Atrial flutter
- Associated with hydrops
- Both confer poor prognosis

Treatment
- If pregnancy termination: Encourage autopsy
- Not indication for karyotype if isolated
- Pediatric cardiology consult
- Monitor for arrythmia
- Monitor for hydrops
  - o **Early delivery does not improve prognosis**
  - o Consider maternal digitalization for fetal tachycardia
- Deliver at tertiary center

Prognosis
- Fetal diagnosis
  - o 48% intrauterine fetal demise
  - o 10% survive neonatal period
  - o Poor prognostic indicators: Predict death by 3 months
    - ▪ Tethered anterosuperior leaflet
    - ▪ Left ventricular compression
    - ▪ Right ventricular dysplasia
- Live born postnatal diagnosis: Asymptomatic to severe cyanosis at birth depending on
  - o Degree RV obstruction
  - o Degree of tricuspid displacement
  - o Overall 67% survival at 1 year, 59% at 10 years
- Surgery: TV repair/replacement
  - o Prenatal/early diagnosis ⇒ most severe cases ⇒ worst outcome
- Recurrence risk
  - o One child 1%
  - o Two affected 3%

Selected References
1. Hsieh YY et al: Successful prenatal digoxin therapy for Ebstein's anomaly with hydrops fetalis. J Reprod Med 43:710-12, 1998
2. Hornberger LK et al: Tricuspid valve disease with significant tricuspid insufficiency in the fetus: Diagnosis and outcome. J Am Coll Cardiol 17:167-73, 1991
3. Sharland GK et al: Tricuspid valve dysplasia or displacement in intrauterine life. J Am Coll Cardiol 15:944-9, 1991

Pulmonary Atresia

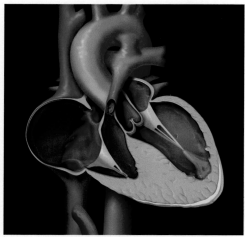

Pulmonary atresia. Diagram depicts membranous occlusion of the pulmonary valve. RV and PA are hypoplastic. There is reversed flow in the ductus arteriosus.

Key Facts
- Definition: Obstruction to right ventricular outflow tract (RVOT) at level of pulmonary valve (PV)
- Classic imaging appearance: **Absent antegrade flow across pulmonary valve**
- Valve may be
  - Completely absent: Muscular atresia
  - Present but occluded by membrane
- Range of appearances
  - 23%: Pulmonary atresia (PA) with intact ventricular septum (IVS)
    - May progress to hypoplastic right heart (HRH) physiology
  - 46%: PA with ventriculoseptal defect (VSD)
    - Tetralogy of Fallot physiology (PA/VSD)
  - 31%: PA + additional complex cardiac malformation

Imaging Findings
<u>General Features</u>
- Best imaging clue: No antegrade flow across pulmonary valve
  - Aortic valve (AV) and PV are always side by side
<u>Ultrasound Findings</u>
- **Right atrial enlargement**
  - Blood cannot exit right ventricle (RV) antegrade
  - Tricuspid regurgitation ⇒ volume load to right atrium (RA)
- RVOT abnormally small or not identified
- **Retrograde flow in ductus arteriosus**
- **PA/IVS subtype**
  - **Obliteration of RV cavity over time**
  - Blood "must" get out ⇒ coronary artery fistula
  - Abnormal 4-chamber view
    - RV << left ventricle (LV)
    - RA enlarged

Pulmonary Atresia

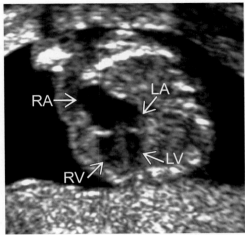

Pulmonary atresia. 4-chamber view in 17 week fetus with pulmonary atresia and intact ventricular septum. The RA is markedly enlarged due to tricuspid regurgitation. The RV is normal at this point but would ultimately become hypoplastic. Note abnormal cardiac axis. RVOT could not be identified.

- **PA/VSD subtype**
  - ○ Flow across VSD ⇒ ventricles symmetric
  - ○ "Large" aorta: Receives blood from both ventricles

Imaging Recommendations
- Formal fetal echocardiography
  - ○ RV-coronary artery fistula
    - ▪ Distal RV-R coronary artery
    - ▪ Bidirectional arterial flow
    - ▪ Courses along outer wall of heart
  - ○ Ductus diameter decreased (2-4 mm)
    - ▪ Normal growth ⇒ linear increase in diameter
  - ○ Other cardiac anomalies
    - ▪ Heterotaxia
    - ▪ Tricuspid atresia
    - ▪ Transposition great vessels
- Careful search for noncardiac anomalies

Differential Diagnosis

Hypoplastic Left Heart
- LV < RV
  - ○ RV is anterior ventricle
- Left ventricular outflow track (LVOT)/aorta small
  - ○ RVOT is anterior
  - ○ Branches into ductus/right pulmonary artery (RPA) shortly after exiting the heart

Tetralogy of Fallot
- Pulmonary infundibular stenosis is typical lesion
  - ○ Pulmonary atresia can occur
- VSD must be present: VSD not part of PA/IVS

Pulmonary Atresia

Pathology

General

- General Path Comments
  - Associated with stenosis of pulmonary artery and branches
  - Associated with abnormal ductus arteriosus connections
    - Aortic origin more proximal
    - Pulmonary artery origin from branch, not main
- Genetics
  - Case reports of siblings: Possible autosomal recessive
  - 22q11 deletion more common in PA/VSD
    - Velocardiofacial syndrome
    - Dysmorphic features
    - Cardiac malformations
- Epidemiology
  - PA/IVS 4.2:100,000 live births in Sweden
  - All types 21.4:100,000 live births in UK

Clinical Issues

Presentation

- PA/IVS with RV-coronary fistula reported at 17 weeks (EV scans)

Natural History PA/IVS

- Severe hypoxia at birth
  - Cardiomegaly $\Rightarrow$ pulmonary hypoplasia
  - Heart failure

Treatment

- Genetic counseling: Offer karyotype
- Prenatal consultation with pediatric cardiologist
- Deliver at tertiary care facility
  - 4/5 "maternally" transported cases survived intervention
- Ductus dependent pulmonary circulation
- **Ductal closure is life threatening**
  - Avoid maternal prostaglandin administration

Prognosis

- PA/IVS
  - 90% require surgery within first week of life
- PA/VSD
  - > 50% require surgery within 1 month
  - > 25% require surgery within 3 months
- Surgical mortality 23%
- Total mortality in first year 38%
- Poor prognostic markers
  - Low birth weight
  - Male gender
  - Muscular pulmonary atresia

Selected References
1. Nishibatake M et al: Echocardiographic findings of pulmonary atresia or critical pulmonary stenosis and intact ventricular septum in utero. Pediatr Int 41:716-21, 1999
2. Chaoui R et al: Prenatal diagnosis of ventriculo-coronary communication in a second-trimester fetus using transvaginal and transabdominal color Doppler sonography. Ultrasound Obstet Gynecol 9:194-7, 1997
3. Marino B et al: Ductus arteriosus in pulmonary atresia with and without ventricular septal defect. Scan J Thorac Cardiovasc Surg 26:93-6, 1992

PocketRadiologist®
Obstetrics
Top 100 Diagnoses

ABDOMINAL WALL

Omphalocele

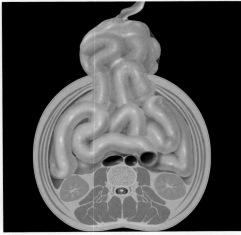

Omphalocele. Illustration shows a midline abdominal wall defect with herniation of small bowel. It is covered by a membrane with the umbilical cord inserting directly on the mass.

Key Facts

- Definition: Midline abdominal wall defect with herniation of abdominal contents into base of umbilical cord
- Classic imaging appearance: Smooth, well-circumscribed mass protruding from an abdominal wall defect with umbilical cord insertion on mass
- **60-80% have associated structural abnormality**
  o Cardiac most common
- **50% have chromosomal abnormalities**
- Those with **small bowel highest association of aneuploidy**
  o Trisomy 18 most common
- Physiologic bowel herniation until 11.2 weeks
  o Herniated **liver never normal**

Imaging Findings

General Features
- Best imaging clue: Color Doppler shows **umbilical cord insertion on mass**
- Liver and small bowel most common contents
  o Spleen, bladder, stomach, and large bowel also reported

Ultrasound Findings
- Smooth, **central** abdominal mass
- Umbilical cord inserts on sac
- Polyhydramnios common
- Ascites may be present
- Associated structural abnormalities
  o **Cardiac defects**
  o GI: Congenital diaphragmatic hernia, atresias, malrotation
  o Umbilical cord cysts
- Syndromes
  o OEIS Complex

Omphalocele

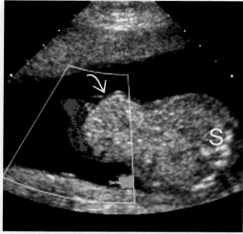

Omphalocele. Axial image of the fetal abdomen shows a large central abdominal wall defect with herniation of liver and bowel. It is covered by a smooth membrane (arrow) with umbilical cord inserting centrally on the mass. (S - spine).

- Omphalocele
- Exstrophy
- Imperforate anus
- Spine abnormalities
o Beckwith-Wiedemann syndrome
  - Omphalocele
  - Hemihypertrophy
  - Organomegaly
  - Macroglossia
o Pentalolgy of Cantrell
  - Omphalocele
  - Ectopia cordis
  - Cardiac anomalies
  - Sternal, pericardial, diaphragmatic defects

MR Findings
- Useful in obese patients for differentiating contents of sac
- SSFSE: Liver – low signal, bowel contents – serpiginous high signal

Imaging Recommendations
- Careful search for other abnormalities
- Dedicated cardiac echo

Differential Diagnosis

Gastroschisis
- Cord inserts on abdominal wall
- No covering membrane
- Free floating loops of bowel
- Does not contain liver

Body Stalk Anomaly
- Fetus adherent to placenta
- No free floating umbilical cord

Omphalocele

- Scoliosis

Bladder/Cloacal Exstrophy
- Umbilical cord inserts above defect
- Absent bladder is hallmark

Physiologic Gut Herniation
- Bowel returns to abdomen by 11.2 weeks
- Should not extend more than 1 cm
- Never contains liver

Pathology
General
- Genetics
  o Most sporadic
  o Chromosomal abnormalities
    ▪ **Trisomy 18**, Trisomy 13, Triploidy, Turner syndrome (45X)
- Embryology: Proposed mechanisms
  o Liver containing: Failure of body wall closure
  o Bowel containing: Persistence of body stalk
- Epidemiology
  o 1:4,000 births
  o Incidence increases with **advanced maternal age**

Gross Pathologic, Surgical Features
- Mass **covered by both peritoneum and amnion** with Wharton's jelly in between

Clinical Issues
Presentation
- Elevated maternal serum alpha-fetoprotein (70%)

Natural History
- In utero rupture rare
  o Difficult to differentiate from gastroschisis
- Small omphaloceles
  o Often just small bowel
  o Higher association with structural and chromosomal anomalies
- Giant omphaloceles
  o Large abdominal wall defect
  o Small chest → pulmonary hypoplasia

Treatment
- **Amniocentesis for karyotype**
- Delivery at tertiary care facility
- Benefits of cesarean section controversial
  o Not indicated if multiple associated anomalies
- Surgical or gradual (pressure) reduction based on size

Prognosis
- Survival as high as 80-90% if normal chromosomes, no other anomalies
- Associated structural or chromosomal abnormalities **mortality 80-100%**

Selected References
1. Snijders RJ et al: Fetal exomphalos at 11 to 14 weeks of gestation. J Ultrasound Med 14:569-74, 1995
2. Hughes MD et al: Fetal omphalocele: Prenatal US detection of concurrent anomalies and other predictors of outcome. Radiology 173:371-6, 1989
3. Nyberg DA et al: Chromosomal abnormalities in fetuses with omphalocele. Significance of omphalocele contents. J Ultrasound Med 8:299-308, 1989

Gastroschisis

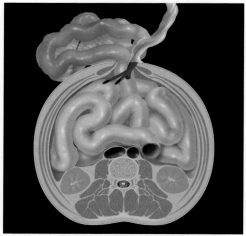

Gastroschisis. Illustration shows an abdominal wall defect with herniation of small bowel. The defect is adjacent to the normally inserting umbilical cord.

Key Facts
- Definition: Bowel herniation through a paramedian abdominal wall defect
- Classic imaging appearance: **Free floating loops of bowel** adjacent to a normally inserting umbilical cord
- Associated GI abnormalities
  - **Malrotation > 95%**
  - Atresias 5-30%
- Almost invariably on **right**
- More common in **young women**
- Not associated with chromosomal abnormalities

Imaging Findings
General Features
- Best imaging clue: Color Doppler shows **umbilical cord insertion in normal location**
- Herniated contents generally small bowel
  - Large bowel and stomach also reported
Ultrasound Findings
- **No covering membrane**
- **Bowel wall may become thickened, echogenic, and nodular**
  - Secondary to edema and fibrinous serosal deposits
- Bowel dilatation
  - Both intra- and extra-abdominal loops may be dilated
  - Greater dilatation, poorer prognosis
- Stomach often malpositioned
- Oligohydramnios more common than polyhydramnios
  - Polyhydramnios suggests associated atresia
- Intrauterine growth restriction (IUGR) common
Imaging Recommendations
- Document cord insertion with **normal abdominal wall on both sides**
  - May miss if incompletely evaluated

Gastroschisis

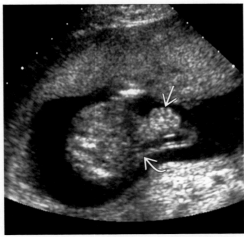

Gastroschisis. Axial image through the abdomen of a 17 week fetus shows herniation of small bowel (arrow) adjacent to a normally inserting umbilical cord (curved arrow).

- Close US follow-up for fetal distress
  - Progressive bowel dilatation
  - Developing IUGR
    - Abdominal circumference is small making evaluation difficult
  - Oligohydramnios

Differential Diagnosis
Omphalocele
- **Cord inserts on mass**
- Covered by peritoneum
- Ruptured omphalocele difficult to differentiate
  - Consider if liver present
  - Rare

Body Stalk Anomaly
- Fetus adherent to placenta
- No free floating umbilical cord
- Scoliosis

Bladder/Cloacal Exstrophy
- Umbilical cord inserts above defect
- Absent bladder is hallmark

Physiologic Gut Herniation
- Bowel returns to abdomen by 11.2 weeks
- Should not extend more than 1 cm
- Always midline

Pathology
General
- Association with non-GI abnormalities low
- Genetics
  - Most are sporadic

Gastroschisis

- o Familial cases reported
    - ▪ 3.5% recurrence risk
- o No chromosomal associations
    - ▪ Amniocentesis not indicated
- Embryology: Proposed mechanisms
    - o **Abnormal involution of right umbilical vein**
    - o Vascular accident involving omphalomesenteric artery (less likely)
- Epidemiology
    - o 1:3,000 births
    - o Incidence increasing

Gross Pathologic, Surgical Features
- Defect relatively small (< 5 cm)
- Exposed loops inflamed and edematous
- Atresias often present

Clinical Issues
Presentation
- Elevated maternal serum alpha-fetoprotein (95%)
    - o Exposed bowel results in greater elevations than with omphalocele
Natural History
- May resorb on follow-up exam ("vanishing gut")
    - o Associated with tight defects
        - ▪ Ischemia → infarction → atresia (often long segment)
- **Premature delivery common**
- **Bowel complications** much greater than for omphalocele
    - o Amniotic fluid irritating leading to atresias, edema, poor function
Treatment
- Amnioinfusion may improve outcome (experimental studies)
    - o Decreases concentration of irritants in amniotic fluid
- Delivery at tertiary care center
- Early delivery considered if worsening bowel dilatation (controversial)
- Cesarean section common but value is questioned
- Immediate surgical repair
    - o Large defects may require delayed secondary fascial closure
- Parenteral nutrition post-op until intestinal function returns
    - o May require several weeks
Prognosis
- **90% survival**
    - o Deaths from prematurity, sepsis, or bowel complications
- 10-15% persistent disability
    - o Motility disorders
    - o Short gut syndrome

Selected References
1. Luton D et al: Effect of amnioinfusion on the outcome of prenatally diagnosed gastroschisis. Fetal Diagn Ther 14:152-5, 1999
2. Adra AM et al: The fetus with gastroschisis: Impact of route of delivery and prenatal ultrasonography. Am J Obstet Gynecol 174:540-6, 1996
3. Babcook CJ et al: Gastroschisis: can sonography of the fetal bowel accurately predict postnatal outcome? J Ultrasound Med 13:701-6, 1994

Body Stalk Anomaly

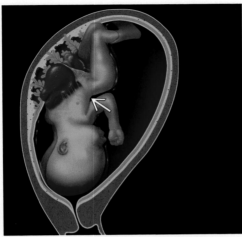

Body stalk anomaly. Drawing depicts fetus anchored to placenta by abdominal wall defect. Liver and bowel are involved in the defect. Fetal peritoneum is in continuity with amnion. Scoliosis (arrow) results from fetal tethering.

Key Facts
- Synonyms: Limb body wall complex, body stalk complex, cyllosomas
- Definition: Open abdominal wall defect with fetal peritoneum in continuity with amniotic cavity
- Classic imaging appearance
  o Abdominal wall defect (AWD)
  o Fetus "tethered" to placenta at defect
  o Scoliosis
- Umbilical cord absent or very short

Imaging Findings
General Features
- Best imaging clue: Abdominal wall defect with fetus adherent to placenta
Ultrasound Findings
- No membrane covering defect
- No umbilical cord insertion site
- Absent/very short umbilical cord
  o Vessels seen running from placental surface to fetal torso
- Scoliosis
  o Often severe
- Abnormal limb positioning
- Neck often extended
Imaging Recommendations
- Fixed fetal/placental relationship essential for diagnosis
  o Scan mother in different positions
  o Have mother walk, eat, return later in day

Differential Diagnosis
Gastroschisis
- **Mobile** fetus

Body Stalk Anomaly

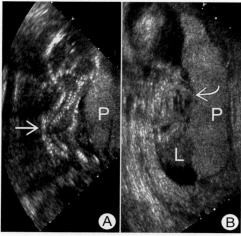

Body stalk anomaly. Ultrasound images depict scoliosis (arrow). The abdominal wall defect includes the heart and liver (L). Both the heart (curved arrow) and the liver were adherent to the placenta (P).

- Normal cord: Inserts **beside** defect which is usually small
- Defect not covered: Bowel floats free in amniotic fluid

Omphalocele
- **Mobile** fetus
- Normal cord: Inserts on **apex** of defect
- Membrane covered

Bladder/Cloacal Exstrophy
- **Mobile** fetus
- Normal cord: Inserts **above** defect
- Absent bladder is the hallmark

OEIS Complex
- Omphalocele
- Exstrophy (bladder)
- Imperforate anus
- Spine abnormalities
- **Mobile fetus**

Amniotic Band Sequence
- Fetus may be **immobile**
- Normal cord
  - Cord insertion site may be involved if abdominoschisis
- Variable pattern of defects
- Scoliosis not common
- Bands seen in amniotic fluid, may extend to immobile fetal part

Pathology
General
- Genetics
  - Nonhereditary
- Embryology

138

- o Malfunction of the ectodermal placodes involving cephalic and caudal embryonic folding process
- o Malformation of the anterior abdominal wall
- o Malformation of the lateral abdominal wall
- o Body stalk/yolk stalk fusion fails: No umbilical cord
- o Amnion/chorion fusion fails
- o Amnion does not cover cord
- o Amnion in continuity with peritoneum at edge of defect
- Epidemiology
  - o Reported incidence 1:7,500-42,000 in UK
  - o 0.33:1,000 live births in Australia
  - o Associated with
    - Alcohol, tobacco, marijuana use
    - History of prior child with congenital anomaly (any) in 40%

Gross Pathologic, Surgical Features

- AWD with evisceration of organs
- Malformed cord incompletely covered in amnion
- Umbilical vessels embedded in amniotic sheet connecting to skin margin of AWD

Clinical Issues

Presentation

- Abnormal maternal serum screen
  - o Marked elevation maternal serum alpha-fetoprotein
- Can be diagnosed by end first trimester
  - o Normal cord can be identified as early as 8 weeks
  - o Crown-rump length (CRL):Cord length = 1:1
  - o Normal bowel rotation process complete by 11.2 weeks

Treatment

- Amniocentesis not required
  - o No abnormal karyotype reported
- Offer termination
  - o Aim for delivery of intact fetus for autopsy
- Psychological support to family

Prognosis

- Lethal
- Frequent spontaneous abortion

Selected References
1. Luehr B: Limb body wall complex: A case series. J Matern Fetal Neonatal Med 12:132-7, 2002
2. Pumberger W et al: Limb body wall complex: A compound anomaly pattern in body wall defects. Pediatr Surg Int 17:486-90, 2001
3. Colpaert C: Limb body wall complex: 4 new cases illustrating the importance of examining placenta and umbilical cord. Pathol Res Pract 196:783-90, 2000

PocketRadiologist®
Obstetrics
Top 100 Diagnoses

GI

Esophageal Atresia

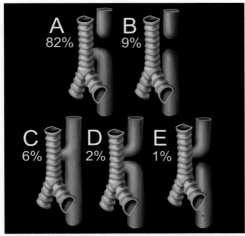

Types of esophageal atresia (EA) in order of descending frequency. (A) EA with distal fistula. (B) EA with no fistula. (C) "H" fistula with no EA. (D) EA with proximal and distal fistula. (E) EA with proximal fistula.

Key Facts

- Definition: Atresia of esophagus often associated with tracheoesophageal fistula (TEF)
- Classic imaging appearance: Small or absent stomach with polyhydramnios
- Proximal esophageal atresia (EA) with distal TEF most common
  - **Stomach may be present** but small
- Associated **malformations in 50-70%**
- Increased risk of Trisomy 18 and 21 (T18, T21)
- Intrauterine growth restriction **(IUGR) common**
  - Ingested fluid plays role in fetal nutrition
- **Polyhydramnios** does not develop until **after 20 weeks**

Imaging Findings

General Features
- Best imaging clue: Combination of small stomach, polyhydramnios, and IUGR in late 2nd and 3rd trimester fetus
  - **Diagnosis often missed** before polyhydramnios develops
    - Reported sensitivity of US for detection of EA < 50%

Ultrasound Findings
- Small or absent stomach
- **"Pouch" sign**
  - Transient filling of proximal esophagus with swallowing
- Frequently associated with duodenal atresia
  - If TEF not present, fluid may accumulate in distal esophagus, stomach, and duodenum forming a **"C" loop**
  - Accumulated secretions may cause marked dilatation
  - High risk for T21
- Part of **VACTERL** association
  - Vertebral anomalies

Esophageal Atresia

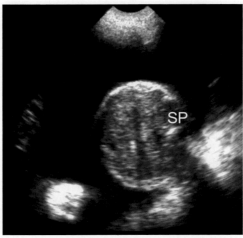

Esophageal atresia. Transverse image of the abdomen in a 26 week fetus shows no stomach bubble. Also note there is marked polyhydramnios. (SP – spine).

o Anal atresia
o Cardiac malformation
o Tracheo-Esophgeal fistula
o Renal anomalies
o Limb malformation

Imaging Recommendations
- Follow-up scans on all fetuses with small stomach
  o May be transient finding in normal fetus especially in 1st and 2nd trimester
- Monitor for polyhydramnios and growth
- Evaluate for other anomalies

Differential Diagnosis
Diaphragmatic Hernia
- Stomach in chest
- Abdominal circumference small
Abnormal Swallowing
- CNS malformations
- Neuromuscular disorders
- Cleft lip, palate

Pathology
General
- General Path Comments
  o Other bowel malformations common
    ▪ Multiple atresias: Duodenal, ileal, anorectal
    ▪ Malrotation
- Genetics
  o Sporadic
- Chromosomal
  o **Trisomy 18** (more common) and 21

144

o EA without TEF more common in T21
- Embryology
  o Failure of tracheoesophageal septum to separate dorsal and ventral foregut
- Epidemiology
  o 1:2,000-3,000 live births

Clinical Issues

Presentation
- Abnormal triple screen (T18, T21)
- Polyhydramnios
  o Large-for-dates
  o Preterm labor
- After delivery
  o Coughing, drooling, choking
  o Recurrent pneumonia (H-type)

Treatment
- All fetuses should be karyotyped
- Surgical resection and reanastomosis after delivery
  o May need to be staged procedure if atretic segment is long
- Gastrostomy tube in some cases

Prognosis
- 25-75% mortality for those detected in utero
- Even if isolated, long-term sequelae common
  o Esophageal dysmotility in nearly 100%
  o Strictures
  o Recurrent TEF
  o Aspiration
  o Feeding difficulties
  o Tracheomalacia

Selected References

1. Sparey C et al: Esophageal atresia in the Northern Region Congenital Anomaly Survey, 1985-1997: Prenatal diagnosis and outcome. Am J Obstet Gynecol 182:427-31, 2000
2. Satoh S et al: Antenatal sonographic detection of the proximal esophageal segment: Specific evidence for congenital esophageal atresia. J Clin Ultrasound 23:419-23, 1995
3. Stringer MD et al: Prenatal diagnosis of esophageal atresia. J Pediatr Surg 30:1258-63, 1995

Duodenal Atresia

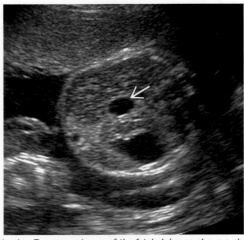

Duodenal atresia. Transverse image of the fetal abdomen shows a classic "double bubble" appearance. (Arrow – duodenum).

Key Facts
- Definition: Lack of normal duodenal canalization leading to partial (web) or complete obstruction (atresia)
- Classic imaging appearance: Dilatation of both stomach and duodenum ("**double bubble**")
- **30% have Down syndrome** (T21)
- **50% have structural abnormalities** including skeletal, cardiac, and GI

Imaging Findings
General Features
- Best imaging clue: **Stomach and duodenum can be connected** during real-time imaging
- Normal gastric incisura may mimic appearance
- Fluid in duodenum is always abnormal
Ultrasound Findings
- "Double bubble"
  - Generally seen after 20 weeks
  - Seen earlier in select cases
    - May have worse prognosis
- **Polyhydramnios** may become severe
  - Usually not detected before 24 weeks
- No fluid in distal bowel loops
- Fetal regurgitation may intermittently decompress stomach
- Other GI malformations common
  - Esophageal atresia 7%
    - If tracheoesophageal fistula (TEF) not present, fluid may accumulate in distal esophagus, stomach, and duodenum forming a **"C" loop**
    - Accumulated secretions may cause marked dilatation
    - **High risk for T21**
  - Distal bowel atresia

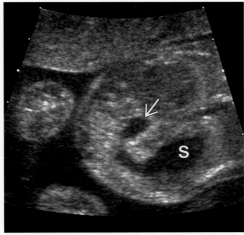

Duodenal atresia. An angled view in the same fetus shows communication between these two "fluid collections" confirming the diagnosis of duodenal atresia. (S – stomach, arrow – duodenum).

- o Malrotation
- o Biliary atresia
- Other associated findings
  - o Cardiac
    - Atrioventricular septal defect (AVSD)
    - **AVSD + duodenal atresia (DA) greatest risk of T21**
  - o Skeletal
    - Vertebral body malformations
    - Radial ray malformation
    - Sacral agenesis
    - Clubfeet
  - o GU
    - Hydronephrosis
    - Multicystic dysplastic kidney

Imaging Recommendations
- Look for findings of T21
- Dedicated cardiac echo
- Follow for worsening polyhydramnios

Differential Diagnosis
Abdominal Cysts
- **None will communicate with stomach**
- Polyhydramnios not a feature
- Choledochal cyst
  - o Right-sided near gallbladder
- Duplication cyst
  - o Duodenal duplication can be difficult
  - o Most more distal
- Ovarian cyst
  - o Female only

o Not usually seen until 3rd trimester

Pathology
General
- Genetics
  o Sporadic
- Chromosomal
  o 30% have T21
  o 15% of T21 have DA
- Embryology: 2 theories
  o Failure of normal recanalization of duodenal lumen at 6-9 weeks
  o Vascular compromise to developing gut
- Epidemiology
  o 1-3:10,000 births
Gross Pathologic, Surgical Features
- 2nd and 3rd portions most commonly involved
- Most near ampulla of Vater
- May be incomplete (web)
  o Same risk of T21
- Annular pancreas frequently present

Clinical Issues
Presentation
- Abnormal triple screen (T21)
- Polyhydramnios
  o Large-for-dates
  o Preterm labor
Treatment
- All fetuses should be karyotyped
- Genetic counseling
- Immediate NG suction after delivery
- Surgical correction in immediate neonatal period
Prognosis
- Dependent on associated abnormalities
- Overall mortality 15%
- Isolated defect 95% survival
- Recurrence risk same as general population

Selected References
1. Lawrence MJ et al: Congenital duodenal obstruction: Early antenatal ultrasound diagnosis. Pediatr Surg Int 16:342-5, 2000
2. Estroff JA et al: Second trimester prenatal findings in duodenal and esophageal atresia without tracheoesophageal fistula. J Ultrasound Med 13:375-9, 1994
3. Grosfeld JL et al: Duodenal atresia and stenosis: Reassessment of treatment and outcome based on antenatal diagnosis, pathologic variance, and long-term follow-up. World J Surg 17:301-9, 1993

Jejunal/Ileal Atresia

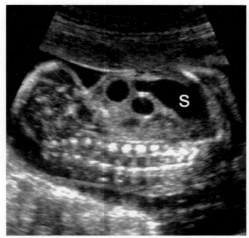

Jejunal atresia. Sagittal ultrasound image in a second trimester fetus shows dilatation of two loops of bowel in addition to the stomach (triple bubble). (S – stomach).

Key Facts
- Definition: One or more areas of stenosis or atresia involving small bowel
- Classic imaging appearance: Dilated loops of bowel and polyhydramnios
- Equal frequency in jejunum and ileum
- **1/3 have cystic fibrosis**
- Extraintestinal anomalies uncommon
  - Atresia in other areas (esophagus, duodenum, anal) much more likely to have associated abnormalities
- **5-10% will perforate** resulting in meconium peritonitis

Imaging Findings
General Features
- Best imaging clue: **Hyperperistalsis** within dilated small bowel loops highly suggestive of obstruction
Ultrasound Findings
- Normal small bowel
  - < 7 mm diameter
  - Seen in 30% after 34 weeks
  - Peristalsis routinely demonstrated
- Atresias
  - **"Triple bubble"** for proximal jejunal atresia
  - **"Sausage-shaped"** bowel loops
  - May not be seen before 26 weeks
  - Polyhydramnios develops in 3rd trimester
  - Hyperperistalsis of obstructed segments
  - Enlarging bowel 3rd trimester
MR Findings
- May better delineate site of obstruction
- Difference in signal characteristics between loops suggests multiple sites of atresia

Jejunal/Ileal Atresia

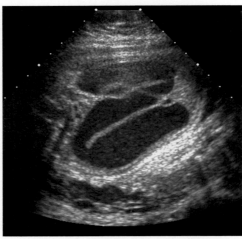

Ileal atresia. An oblique image through the abdomen in a third trimester fetus shows marked dilatation of several loops of bowel creating a "sausage-shaped" appearance.

Imaging Recommendations
- Frequent follow-up scans
  - Growth
    - Proximal atresias more likely to show intrauterine growth restriction (IUGR)
  - Increasing dilatation
  - Polyhydramnios
  - Perforation

Differential Diagnosis
Normal Colon
- 18 mm in 3rd trimester

Meconium Ileus
- Obstruction from meconium impaction in distal ileum
- Often indistinguishable from atresia
- High association with cystic fibrosis
  - Echogenic bowel on 2nd trimester scan

Midgut Volvulus
- Ischemia leads to infarction
  - Dilated bowel segment shows no peristalsis
  - Heterogeneous lumen contents from hemorrhage and necrosis
- May be indistinguishable early

Abdominal Cysts
- Choledochal, duplication, ovarian, mesenteric
  - Single cysts, not tubular
  - Not usually associated with polyhydramnios

Pathology
General
- Frequently associated with other GI malformations

Jejunal/Ileal Atresia

- o Gastroschisis
- o Volvulus
- o Intussusception
- o Malrotation
- Genetics
  - o Sporadic
  - o Familial cases of multiple atresias reported
  - o Cystic fibrosis: Autosomal recessive
    - Gene mutation chromosome 7
    - 25% recurrence risk
- Etiology-Pathogenesis
  - o Vascular injury
    - Kinking of artery during bowel rotation (6-12 weeks)
    - Hypotension
    - Vascular malformation
- Epidemiology
  - o 1:3,000

Gross Pathologic, Surgical Features
- May occur as web, short segment, or long segment ("apple-peel")

Clinical Issues

Presentation
- Dilated bowel and polyhydramnios in 2nd and 3rd trimester
  - o Sensitivity for US detection reported as high as 100%

Natural History
- Ileal
  - o More likely to perforate
- **Jejunal**
  - o **Higher association with premature delivery**
    - Likely secondary to polyhydramnios
  - o **IUGR**
    - Amniotic fluid nutritional source for fetus
  - o More likely to have multiple atresias
    - Not detectable prenatally because segments distal to obstruction are decompressed

Treatment
- Amniocentesis for cystic fibrosis
- Resection and reanastomosis

Prognosis
- > 90% survival
- Negatively impacted by
  - o Increasing length of atretic segment
  - o Multiple sites of atresia
  - o Proximal vs distal

Selected References
1. Corteville JE et al: Bowel abnormalities in the fetus--correlation of prenatal ultrasonographic findings with outcome. Am J Obstet Gynecol 175:724-9, 1996
2. Estroff JA et al: Prevalence of cystic fibrosis in fetuses with dilated bowel. Radiology 183:677-80, 1992
3. Nyberg DA et al: Fetal bowel. Normal sonographic findings. J Ultrasound Med 6:3-6, 1987

Meconium Peritonitis/Pseudocyst

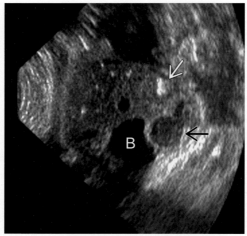

Meconium peritonitis. Fetal US shows calcifications (white arrow), confirmed to be capsular on other scan planes. The bladder (B) is full. Multiple distended bowel loops (black arrow) were seen. No pseudocyst identified in this case.

Key Facts
- Definition: Chemical peritonitis due to intrauterine bowel perforation
- Classic imaging appearance: Dilated bowel loops, peritoneal calcifications, and ascites
- Classified as
  - Simple: Calcifications without bowel abnormality
    - Majority have no adverse outcome
    - Unlikely to require postnatal surgery
  - Complex: Calcifications associated with cyst formation/abnormal bowel
    - Increased risk for postnatal surgery
    - Small series: Surgery rates 22-50%

Imaging Findings
General Features
- Best imaging clue: Intraperitoneal calcifications in 85%
- **Peritoneal calcifications are on liver capsule** not intrahepatic
Ultrasound Findings
- Intraperitoneal calcifications
- Ascites
- Dilated bowel loops
- Cystic mass
- Hydrops
Imaging Recommendations
- Look for calcifications within bowel lumen
  - Presence implies bowel-urinary tract fistula
  - More complex anomaly
- Look for signs of infection
  - Growth restriction
  - Hydrops
  - Intrahepatic (parenchymal) calcifications

Meconium Peritonitis/Pseudocyst

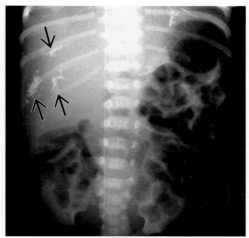

Meconium peritonitis. Postnatal abdominal film of the same infant again shows capsular calcifications (arrows). Ileal atresia was the underlying cause.

  o Intracranial calcifications
- Monitor amniotic fluid
  o Polyhydramnios $\Rightarrow$ preterm labor
- Serial scans through pregnancy
  o Simple may $\Rightarrow$ complex
  o Change impacts delivery plan

Differential Diagnosis
Abdominal Calcifications
- Gallstones
- **Intrahepatic: Infection**
  o Cytomegalovirus (CMV), toxoplasmosis, Parvovirus
- Tumors: Hepatoblastoma, teratoma, neuroblastoma
Ascites
- Hydrops
  o Must have ascites + fluid in one other area
  o Check cardiac structure, rate and rhythm
- Urinary
  o Associated with obstructive uropathy
  o Peristalsing tube that connects to kidney, goes behind bladder or touches spine more likely ureter than bowel
Sacrococcygeal Teratoma
- Type 4 lesions: Entirely internal
  o Rarely cystic
  o Calcifications, if present, are in mass

Pathology
General
- Associated with other GI malformations
  o Gastroschisis
  o Volvulus/intussusception

Meconium Peritonitis/Pseudocyst

- o Bowel atresia/stenosis
- o Hirschsprung disease
- Genetics
  - o Cystic fibrosis (CF)
    - 8% of fetuses
    - 15-40% of postnatal cases
- Etiology-Pathogenesis
  - o Bowel perforation ⇒ meconium spills into peritoneum
  - o Intense inflammatory reaction
  - o Adhesions ⇒ "cyst" formation
  - o Bowel loops may be trapped within "cyst"
  - o Calcifications secondary to inflammation
- Epidemiology
  - o 1:35,000 live births

Clinical Issues

Presentation
- May present as "isolated" echogenic bowel
  - o Most likely in CF population
  - o Follow fetuses with echogenic bowel for subsequent
    - Dilated loops
    - Evidence of perforation
- Intraperitoneal calcifications at routine scan more usual

Treatment
- Genetic counseling
- Consider parental testing for CF
- Prenatal diagnosis CF available if parents are carriers
- **Simple**: Can deliver in non-academic center
  - o Abdominal examination
  - o Abdominal X-ray
  - o If normal child can feed
  - o Very low risk of surgical intervention
- **Complex**: Deliver at tertiary center
  - o Gastrointestinal contrast studies
  - o 22-50% chance of surgery
  - o Usually resection and enterostomy
    - May require parenteral nutrition
- DNA analysis of newborn preferred over sweat tests
  - o Some mutations found in patients with normal sweat tests

Prognosis
- Fetal diagnosis: Mortality 11-14%
  - o Spontaneous in utero closure of perforation
  - o Detects milder cases
- Neonatal diagnosis: Mortality 40-50%
  - o Higher proportion of cases have cystic fibrosis
  - o > 50% mortality if primary bowel obstruction

Selected References
1. Reynolds E et al: Meconium peritonitis. J Perinatol. 20:193-5, 2000
2. Dirkes K et al: The natural history of meconium peritonitis diagnosed in utero. J Pediatr Surg. 30:979-82, 1995
3. Lockwood C et al: Fetal bowel perforation simulating sacrococcygeal teratoma. J Ultrasound Med. 7:227-9, 1988

Echogenic Bowel

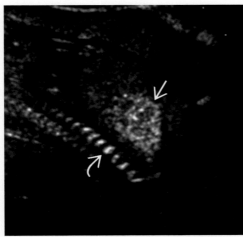

Echogenic bowel. Grade 2 echogenic bowel in a second trimester fetus. Sagittal ultrasound image through the fetal body shows that the fetal bowel (arrow) is as echogenic as the fetal spine (curved arrow).

Key Facts
- Synonyms: Hyperechoic bowel, echogenic abdominal mass
- Definition: Increased echogenicity (whiteness) of fetal bowel during second trimester of pregnancy
- Classic imaging appearance
  - Bowel echogenicity is equal to or greater than that of iliac crest or lumbar spine
- Other key facts
  - As an isolated finding has been associated with multiple other diseases including
    - Increased fetal risk for trisomy 21 (T21)
    - Cystic fibrosis (CF)
    - Cytomegalovirus infection (CMV)
    - Intrauterine growth restriction (IUGR)
    - Intra-amniotic bleeding
  - Seen with other anomalies, associated with increased risk for
    - Trisomy 18
    - Trisomy 13
    - Turner syndrome
  - Echogenic bowel is otherwise seen in 1% of normal obstetrical sonograms

Imaging Findings
General Features
- Best imaging clue
  - During **second trimester, fetal bowel appears focally echogenic** (white), almost mass-like, in fetal lower abdomen & pelvis
Ultrasound Findings
- Bowel echogenicity grading system
  - Grade 0: Bowel echogenicity = liver

Echogenic Bowel

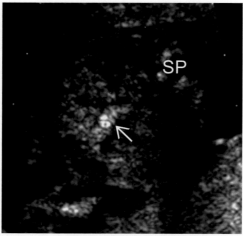

Echogenic bowel. Grade 3 echogenic bowel in a second trimester fetus with trisomy 21. Transverse ultrasound image through fetal pelvis shows focally increased bowel echogenicity (arrow), which is greater than the echogenicity of fetal spine (SP).

- ○ Grade 1: Bowel is mildly echogenic but less than bone
- ○ Grade 2: Bowel is as echogenic as bone
- ○ Grade 3: Bowel echogenicity is greater than bone

Imaging Recommendations
- The more focal and echogenic the bowel, the more abnormal the finding
- **Higher transducer frequency may falsely increase bowel** echogenicity
  - ○ Finding may revert to normal when a lower frequency transducer (≤ 5 MHz) is used
- In order to compare with fetal bone, obtain longitudinal images that include lumbar spine and transverse images that include iliac crest
- Always look for other markers of chromosome aneuploidy
- Refer grade 2 and 3 cases for target exam and genetic counseling

Differential Diagnosis
Normal Bowel
- Grade 0 and 1 are considered normal and are more likely to be diffuse

Normal Third Trimester Colon
- Colonic meconium can normally be seen in third trimester and is not associated with any adverse outcome

Meconium Peritonitis
- Linear and curvilinear calcifications cause increased echogenicities that outline fetal bowel and liver
- Likely to see distended bowel if there is an associated bowel atresia
- May be associated with an increased risk for CF
- Follow-up ultrasound for pseudocyst formation and bowel obstruction but usually finding is idiopathic and without sequelae

Echogenic Bowel

Pathology
General
- Etiology-Suggested Pathogenesis
  - Abnormal low levels of microvillar enzymes in T21 and CF
  - Inspissated meconium
  - Impaired bowel motility with slow transit of bowel contents
  - Mesenteric ischemia
  - Intra-amniotic bleeding with secondary swallowed blood
- Grade 2 and 3 echogenic bowel associated with increased likelihood T21
  - When finding is present, patient is **5.5 x more likely to have a fetus with T21** than her baseline risk based on maternal age and maternal serum screening tests
- Epidemiology
  - Grade 2 or 3 bowel is seen in 1% of fetal population

Clinical Issues
Presentation
- Most cases are isolated, idiopathic, and present at routine obstetrical ultrasound sonogram

Treatment
- Grade 2 and 3 cases need careful sonographic evaluation for additional anomalies and genetic counseling

Prognosis
- Prognosis for Grade 2 and 3 cases as follows
  - 5.5 time increased risk for T21
  - 13% increased risk for CF
  - 18% increased risk for IUGR
  - 62% adverse outcome (isolated and non-isolated cases combined)
  - 35% adverse outcome when isolated

Selected References
1. Nyberg DA et al: Isolated sonographic markers for detection of fetal Down syndrome in the second trimester of pregnancy. J Ultrasound Med 20 (10):1053-63, 2001
2. Slotnick R et al: Prognostic implications of fetal echogenic bowel. Lancet 347:85-7, 1996
3. Nyberg DA et al: Fetal hyperechogenic bowel and Down syndrome. Ultrasound Obstet Gynecol 3:330-3, 1993

Duplication Cyst

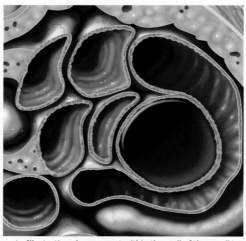

Duplication cyst. Illustration shows a cyst within the wall of the small intestine. Note the thick muscular wall, which is contiguous with the bowel wall. There is mass effect on the intestinal lumen, which can lead to obstruction.

Key Facts
- Synonym: Enteric duplication cyst
- Definition: Abnormal canalization of alimentary tract resulting in duplicated segments occurring in 2 forms
  - Cystic 80%
  - Tubular 20%
- Classic imaging appearance: Cystic abdominal mass
- May cause bowel obstruction
- 40% involve ileum

Imaging Findings
General Features
- Best imaging clue: Thick-walled cyst with hyperechoic lining and layered appearance **(gut signature)**
  - Often difficult to discern
  - Focused high-resolution images needed
- Tubular duplications communicate with bowel and are usually not detected in utero
- Peristalsis within cyst has been described
- Difficult to differentiate from other cystic abdominal masses
Ultrasound Findings
- Generally anechoic but can be echogenic
- Findings vary according to location
  - Small bowel
    - Solitary abdominal cyst
  - Stomach
    - Appears as **cyst within gastric lumen**
  - Esophagus
    - Mediastinal cyst

Duplication Cyst

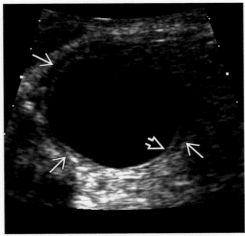

Duplication cyst in a second trimester fetus. A focused, high resolution image of an abdominal cyst shows a thick wall with a layered appearance (arrows). Note the hyperechoic mucosal lining (open arrow).

- Vertebral anomalies commonly associated especially **hemivertebrae**
- Rarely bowel dilatation from obstruction
  - Polyhydramnios may develop

MR Findings
- Well-defined high-signal mass on T2WI

Imaging Recommendations
- Confirm cyst is intraperitoneal and separate from urinary tract
  - **Most cystic abdominal masses are related to urinary tract**
- Obtain enlarged, high-resolution images looking at wall thickness and morphology
- Follow for enlargement or bowel obstruction
  - Polyhydramnios may develop

Differential Diagnosis

Ovarian Cyst
- Females only
- Not seen until 3rd trimester
- Most common abdominal cystic mass in female

Mesenteric Cyst
- Thinner wall
- Less likely to cause obstruction
- Appearance may be identical
- Much less common

Choledochal Cyst
- Right upper quadrant
- Associated with liver

Meconium Pseudocyst
- Often irregular contour
- Wall can calcify

- Other sequelae of meconium peritonitis
  - Peritoneal calcifications
  - Dilated bowel

Dilated Bowel
- Tubular appearance
- Contents echogenic (succus entericus)
- Peristalsis confirmatory

Urachal Cyst
- Midline
- Between dome of bladder and cord insertion

Hydrocolpos
- Midline pelvic mass
- Posterior to bladder
- Not seen until 3rd trimester

Pathology
General
- Embryology: 2 theories
  - Abnormal recanalization
    - Alimentary tract begins as solid tube
    - Normal lumen forms from coalescence of developing vacuoles
    - Duplication occurs if vacuoles split into 2 groups with a dividing septum
  - Abnormal separation from notochord
    - Explains association of esophageal duplication and vertebral abnormalities

Gross Pathologic, Surgical Features
- Occurs on mesenteric side of bowel
- Has a muscular wall

Clinical Issues
Presentation
- In utero
  - Incidental finding
    - Reported as early as 12 weeks
  - May cause bowel obstruction
- Most present in childhood
  - Intussusception
  - Bleeding

Treatment
- Workup after delivery to confirm diagnosis
- Surgical resection

Prognosis
- Excellent

Selected References
1. Chen M et al: Sonographic features of ileal duplication cyst at 12 weeks. Prenat Diagn 22:1067-70, 2002
2. Richards DS et al: The prenatal sonographic appearance of enteric duplication cysts. Ultrasound Obstet Gynecol 7:17-20, 1996
3. Bidwell JK et al: Prenatal ultrasonic diagnosis of congenital duplication of the stomach. J Ultrasound Med 5:589-91, 1986

Choledochal Cyst

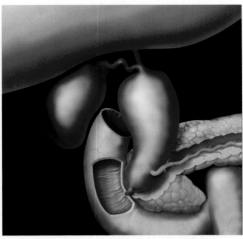

Choledochal cyst. Illustration shows marked dilatation of the common bile duct. Note the anomalous pancreatico-biliary junction with the pancreatic duct inserting into the common bile duct proximal to the sphincter of Oddi.

Key Facts
- Definition: Congenital cystic dilatation of extrahepatic and/or intrahepatic bile ducts
- Classic imaging appearance: Cystic right upper quadrant (RUQ) mass
- Associated with an **anomalous pancreatico-biliary junction (APBJ)**
- Can lead to liver failure if untreated
- Risk factor for cholangiocarcinoma

Imaging Findings
General Features
- Best imaging clue: **Following bile ducts into cyst confirms diagnosis**
  - May be difficult to see
Ultrasound Findings
- Simple cystic mass in RUQ
- Variable size
  - May be large
- Difficult to differentiate from other cystic abdominal masses
MR Findings
- Limited experience
- T2WI to evaluate bile ducts
- MR cholangiogram may prove helpful
Imaging Recommendations
- Confirm position of gallbladder
  - Cyst generally adjacent
- Follow liver contour
  - Immediately adjacent to capsule
  - Coronal view most helpful
    - Subhepatic

Choledochal Cyst

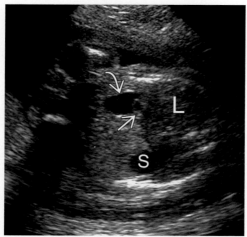

Choledochal cyst in a 26 week fetus. Oblique coronal sonogram of the fetal abdomen shows a large cystic mass subjacent to the inferior margin of the liver (curved arrow). It is immediately adjacent to the gallbladder (white arrow). (L-liver, S-stomach).

Differential Diagnosis
Gallbladder Duplication
- Same fusiform shape as normal gallbladder

Liver Cyst
- Within liver parenchyma

Enteric Duplication Cyst
- Located anywhere in abdomen
  - Ileum most common

Mesenteric Cyst
- Located anywhere in abdomen

Duodenal Atresia
- Connects to stomach in oblique plain

Ovarian Cyst
- Females only
- Seen in 3rd trimester

Meconium Pseudocyst
- Often irregular contour
- Wall can calcify
- Other sequelae of meconium peritonitis
  - Peritoneal calcifications
  - Dilated bowel

Umbilical Vein Varix
- Color Doppler confirms flow

Pathology
General
- Etiology-Pathogenesis: Possible mechanisms (likely multifactorial)

Choledochal Cyst

- o Strong association with APBJ
  - Insertion of pancreatic duct into common bile duct (CBD) above sphincter complex
  - Reflux of pancreatic enzymes into bile duct with weakening of wall
  - Does not completely explain very early cysts
- o Abnormal recanalization during organogenesis
- o Abnormal epithelium resulting in wall weakness
- Epidemiology
  - o Rare in western population
  - o More common in Asia
    - 1/3 of all cases from Japan
  - o F > M

Gross Pathologic, Surgical Features
- Thickened fibrotic wall without epithelial lining

Todani Classification
- **Type 1: Saccular or fusiform dilatation of CBD**
  - o 80-90% of cases
  - o **Type seen in utero**
  - o Subclassified based on portion of CBD involved
- Type 2: CBD diverticulum
- Type 3: Choledochocele
- Type 4: Intrahepatic and extrahepatic dilatation
- Type 5: Intrahepatic dilatation (Caroli disease)

Clinical Issues

Presentation
- Incidental finding in utero
  - o Diagnosed as early as 15 weeks
- Most present in childhood
  - o Jaundice (most common)
  - o Pain
  - o RUQ mass

Natural History
- Untreated leads to **cholestasis, biliary cirrhosis, and eventual liver failure**
- Risk factor for **cholangiocarcinoma**

Treatment
- Complete workup in neonatal period including MRCP and/or ERCP
- Surgical resection with choledocho- or hepaticojejunostomy

Prognosis
- Good with early treatment before irreversible damage

Selected References
1. Redkar R et al: Antenatal diagnosis of congenital anomalies of the biliary tract. J Pediatr Surg 33:700-4, 1998
2. Benhidjeb T et al: Prenatal diagnosis of a choledochal cyst: A case report and review of the literature. Am J Perinatol 13:207-10, 1996
3. Lugo-Vicente HL: Prenatally diagnosed choledochal cysts: Observation or early surgery? J Pediatr Surg 30:1288-90, 1995

PocketRadiologist

Obstetrics
Top 100 Diagnoses

GU

Renal Agenesis

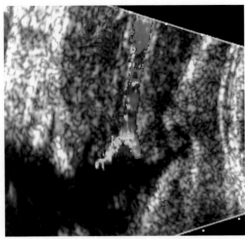

Renal agenesis. Fetal ultrasound with color Doppler of the aorta shows absence of renal arteries. No renal tissue was seen, the bladder was not visualized, and there was anhydramnios.

Key Facts
- Synonym: Potter syndrome
- Definition: Absence of renal tissue
- Classic imaging appearance: **Anhydramnios with failure to demonstrate fetal bladder**
- Bilateral renal agenesis is lethal
- **Diagnosis may be missed in 1st trimester**
- Unilateral agenesis of little concern if solitary kidney normal
- 9% parents/siblings of fetus with bilateral agenesis have asymptomatic renal anomaly
  - Unilateral agenesis
  - Duplication
  - Cystic disease

Imaging Finding
General Features
- Best imaging clue: Anhydramnios, fetal bladder not visible
Ultrasound Findings
- Anhydramnios
- "Absent" bladder
- "Lying down," flattened adrenals
- **Color Doppler**: No demonstrable renal arteries
- Pulmonary hypoplasia
  - Measure cardiac/chest circumference
- 2 vessel cord
- Clubfeet
- Congenital heart disease: 14%
MR Findings
- SSFSE
  - Kidneys/bladder easily visible as early as 15 weeks

Renal Agenesis

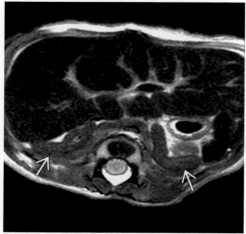

Renal agenesis. Postmortem axial T2WI shows how the adrenals (arrows) occupy the renal fossa and may mimic the presence of kidneys on ultrasound.

  o Not compromised by oligohydramnios
<u>Imaging Recommendations</u>
• Differentiate kidneys from adrenals
  o Adrenals "ice cream sandwich"
    ▪ Hypoechoic cortex
    ▪ Echogenic medulla
• Beware adrenal hypertrophy mimicking presence of kidneys
• Celiac axis, superior mesenteric, adrenal arteries will be present
• Endovaginal scan: Fetal kidneys seen as early as 12 weeks
• Watch for filling and emptying of bladder ⇒ urine production
• Fetal MRI preferable to amnioinfusion for better anatomic visualization

Differential Diagnosis
<u>Premature Rupture of Membranes</u>
• Fetal bladder will fill and empty
• Kidneys present and normal
• Talk to the patient!
<u>Severe Intra-uterine Growth Restriction (IUGR)</u>
• Fetal bladder will fill and empty
• Kidneys present and normal
• Umbilical artery doppler likely abnormal
<u>Sirenomelia</u>
• Bilateral renal agenesis
• Fused lower extremities
• Cardiac/abdominal wall defects
<u>Autosomal Recessive Polycystic Kidneys</u>
• Kidneys present: Enlarged, echogenic
<u>Bilateral Multicystic Dysplastic Kidneys</u>
• Kidneys present: Size variable, visible cysts

Renal Agenesis

Differential Diagnosis for "Absent" Bladder
- No urine formation
- Bladder exstrophy: Urine production $\Rightarrow$ amniotic fluid
- Bladder rupture: Urinary ascites
  - Obstructive nephropathy

Pathology
General
- Genetics
  - Trisomy 7, 10, 21, 22
  - Branchio-oto-renal dysplasia (BOR) syndrome
    - Autosomal dominant: Variable expression
    - Renal anomalies including agenesis
    - Deafness/malformed ears/branchial cysts
  - Cerebro-occulo-facial syndrome
    - Autosomal recessive
    - Micrognathia, joint contractures, renal anomalies
- Embryology
  - Failed induction metanephric blastema by ureteric bud
  - No nephron formation
- Epidemiology
  - Bilateral 1:3,000 births; M>F
  - Unilateral 1:1,300 births

Clinical Issues
Presentation
- **Amniotic fluid volume is normal in first trimester**
  - Renal contribution minimal before 17 weeks
Treatment
- Offer termination
- Psychological support for family
- If pregnancy progresses
  - Do not monitor in labor
  - Stress importance of non-intervention at birth
Prognosis
- Bilateral is lethal: Pulmonary insufficiency
  - 33% stillborn
  - Longest documented survival 39 days
- Unilateral associated with
  - Genital anomalies:
    - Males 12%: Seminal vesicle cysts
    - Females 40%: Mullerian duct anomalies
  - Vesicoureteric reflux in single kidney 30%
  - Increased vesicoureteric/ureteropelvic junction obstruction
- Recurrence risk 3%
  - Higher if part of multiple anomaly complex

Selected References
1. Poutamo J et al: Diagnosing fetal urinary tract anomalies. Acta Obstet Gynecol Scand 79:65-71, 2000
2. Bronshtein M et al: The early prenatal diagnosis of renal agenesis: Techniques and possible pitfalls. Prenat Diagn 14:291-7, 1994
3. McGahan JP et al: Adrenal hypertrophy: Possible pitfall in the sonographic diagnosis of renal agenesis. J Ultrasound Med 5:265-8, 1986

Autosomal Recessive PCKD

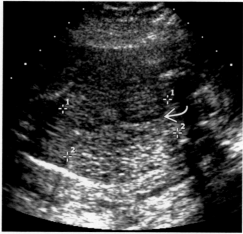

Autosomal recessive PCKD. Coronal US image of an 18 week fetus shows massively enlarged kidneys filling the entire abdomen (cursors). Note the thin hypoechoic rim of normal cortical parenchyma (curved arrow). There is anhydramnios, which impairs visualization.

Key Facts
- Synonym: Infantile polycystic kidney disease
- Definition: Single gene disorder characterized by bilateral symmetric cystic renal disease involving **distal convoluted tubules and collecting ducts**
- Classic imaging appearance: Large echogenic kidneys in a fetus with oligohydramnios
- Kidneys may be large enough to cause dystocia
- **Autosomal recessive ⇒ recurrence risk 25%**

Imaging Findings
<u>General Features</u>
- Best imaging clue: **Enlarged hyperechoic kidneys**
<u>Ultrasound Findings</u>
- Kidneys > 2 SD above mean for gestational age (GA)
  - By late fetal life anywhere from 3–10 x normal size
- Renal enlargement may not occur until mid 2nd trimester
- Cysts may be visible **but do not** predominate
- **Normal hypoechoic cortex is present**
  - Look for thin rim around echogenic medulla
- Oligohydramnios
- Fetal bladder not visible
- Musculoskeletal abnormalities
  - Mechanical: Oligohydramnios limits movement
<u>MR Findings</u>
- SSFSE
  - Large kidneys of uniform high-signal intensity
    - Small, discrete cysts may be discerned
  - No urine in bladder

Autosomal Recessive PCKD

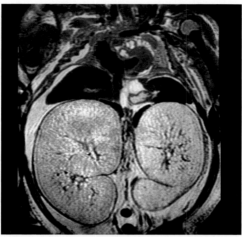

Autosomal recessive PCKD. Postmortem coronal T2WI shows massively enlarged high-signal kidneys. Note small size of thorax due to oligohydramnios and related pulmonary hypoplasia.

<u>Imaging Recommendations</u>
- Serial renal measurements in fetuses at risk
- Ratio renal circumference to abdominal circumference
  - \> 2 SD above mean
- Amniotic fluid assessment
  - 1st or 2nd trimester oligohydramnios ⇒ poor prognosis

Differential Diagnosis
<u>Bilateral Multicystic Dysplastic Kidney</u>
- **Visible macroscopic cysts** dominant feature

<u>Autosomal Dominant Polycystic Kidney Disease</u>
- Check family history and scan parents kidneys
- Asymmetric renal enlargement
- Rare in utero
  - Cysts may be visible late 3rd trimester
- Amniotic fluid normal
- Renal echogenicity normal

<u>Meckel-Gruber</u>
- Encephalocele
  - Microcephaly is a clue if oligohydramnios limits views
- Polydactyly

<u>Trisomy 13</u>
- Kidneys usually small
- Holoprosencephaly
- Polydactyly
- Facial anomalies

<u>Tuberous Sclerosis</u>
- Rhabdomyoma: Echogenic cardiac mass
- Tubers: Subependymal nodules
- Renal cysts not usually seen in utero

Autosomal Recessive PCKD

Beckwith-Wiedemann
- Omphalocele
- Macroglossia
- Gigantism: Often associated polyhydramnios

Pathology
General
- Ectatic distal convoluted tubules and collecting ducts
  - Increased volume of medulla $\Rightarrow$ renal enlargement
  - Increase in reflective interfaces $\Rightarrow$ high echogenicity
- Genetics
  - Autosomal recessive
  - Maps to proximal chromosome 6p
- Epidemiology
  - 1:20,000-50,000 births
  - M=F

Clinical Issues
Presentation
- Majority detected < 24 weeks
  - Diagnosis reported at 16 weeks in at-risk fetus
  - Most kidneys look normal up to 20 weeks
- **May look normal up to late 2nd trimester**
  - Reports of delayed onset oligohydramnios to 28 weeks
Natural History
- **Perinatal form**
  - Severe renal disease
  - Pulmonary hypoplasia
  - Minimal hepatic fibrosis
- **Juvenile form**
  - Minimal renal disease, marked hepatic fibrosis,
  - Liver disease more relevant in survivors
Treatment
- Karyotype
- Deliver at tertiary center
- Monitor abdominal circumference: Risk of dystocia
- Encourage autopsy confirmation if demise or termination
Prognosis
- Fetal diagnosis: Majority stillborn or neonatal death
- Rare survivors will require renal transplant
  - If prolonged survival liver disease becomes relevant
  - Liver transplant currently only available treatment
- Severity and outcomes vary within affected families
- Recurrence risk 25%

Selected References
1. Zerres K et al: Prenatal diagnosis of autosomal recessive polycystic kidney disease (ARPCKD): Molecular genetics, clinical experience and fetal morphology. Am J Med Genet 76:137-44, 1998
2. Barth RA et al: Prenatal diagnosis of autosomal recessive polycystic kidney disease: Variable outcome within one family. Am J Obstet Gynecol 166:560-1, 1992
3. Cohen L et al: Normal length of fetal kidneys. Sonographic study in 397 obstetric patients. AJR 157:545-8 1991

Multicystic Dysplastic Kidney

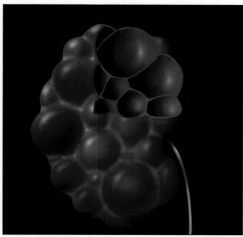

Diagram of multicystic dysplastic kidney showing multiple cysts of varying size with minimal intervening dysplastic tissue.

Key Facts
- Synonym: Mulicystic dysplastic kidney disease (MCDK), renal cystic dysplasia, Potter type II
- Definition: Non-functional renal tissue replaced by multiple cysts and dysplastic tissue
- Classic imaging appearance: **Fetal flank mass with multiple cysts of varying sizes that do not connect**
  - Large cysts distort contour and kidney loses its typical shape
  - Cysts may change size during gestation (may initially enlarge then regress)
- Second most common abdominal mass in a neonate (hydronephrosis #1)
- **40% with contralateral renal abnormalities**
- Can be segmental in duplicated kidneys
- May be associated with other non-renal structural anomalies

Imaging Findings
General Features
- Best imaging clue: Cannot connect the cysts in real-time imaging
Ultrasound Findings
- Paraspinous mass with macroscopic cysts
- Cysts are usually randomly situated, variable in size and shape
- **No normal renal parenchyma is seen**
- May see significant change in cyst size during the pregnancy
- If a bilateral process, may see profound oligohydramnios
Imaging Recommendations
- Careful evaluation of contralateral kidney (40% abnormal)
  - 20% contralateral MCDK (usually fatal)
  - 10% contralateral renal agenesis (usually fatal)
  - 10% contralateral hydronephrosis, usually ureteropelvic junction (UPJ)
- **Follow amniotic fluid volume during pregnancy**
- Careful search for other fetal anomalies

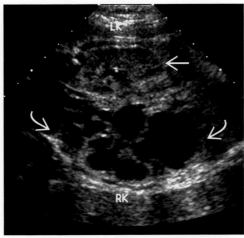

Unilateral multicystic dysplastic kidney. The right kidney (RK, curved arrows) contains multiple cysts of varying sizes. No normal parenchyma is seen. The left kidney (arrow) is normal.

- o **Meckel-Gruber**: MCDK, encephalocele, postaxial polydactyly
- o Trisomy 18, trisomy 13, Jeune syndrome, Zellweger syndrome
- o Genetic counseling/amniocentesis when other anomalies are seen

Differential Diagnosis
Hydronephrosis
- Calyces appear "cyst like" but they communicate with central renal pelvis
Obstructive Uropathy with Renal Dysplasia (Potter Type IV)
- **May appear identical to MCDK if obstruction is early** (before 10 weeks)
- Kidney may keep its reniform shape if obstruction is later
- Sometimes, hydronephrosis seen first with cortical cysts seen later
- Kidney may function if obstruction is late
Autosomal Recessive Polycystic Kidney Disease
- Large echogenic kidneys bilaterally **without** macroscopic cysts
Autosomal Dominant Polycystic Kidney Disease
- Rare in utero
- Echogenic kidneys with few macroscopic cysts and normal fluid
Megaureter: Dilated Ureter
- Usually from obstruction
- Large ureter can be serpiginous and mimic a cystic mass
Congenital Mesoblastic Nephroma
- Solid renal tumor
- Can have cystic necrotic areas

Pathology
General
- Genetics: Not inherited but can be associated with several syndromes
- Etiology-Pathogenesis

Multicystic Dysplastic Kidney

- o Probably due to atresia of ureter or ureteropelvic junction during the metanephric stage of intrauterine development
- o Ureteral atresia prevents metanephric tissue from forming nephrons such that no normal renal parenchyma forms proximally
- o Segmental atresia without renal pelvis atresia leads to more rare hydronephrotic type
- o Atresia of a duplex ureter leads to segmental MCDK
- Epidemiology
  - o M:F = 2:1
  - o 80% are on the left

Gross Pathologic, Surgical Features
- Walls of cysts vary in thickness, fibrotic dysplastic tissue replaces normal renal stroma, may be quite large and non-reniform in shape

Clinical Issues
Presentation
- Incidentally discovered during prenatal ultrasound
- Discovered in infancy as a palpable mass
- Can have delayed presentation as incidental finding when symptoms of contralateral UPJ obstruction are evaluated

Natural History
- Vast majority involute with time and remain asymptomatic
- Can have complications of infection, mass effect, or hypertension

Treatment
- Surgical excision when complicated by focal enlargement (potential Wilms tumor), recurrent infections, mass effect, or hypertension
- Otherwise, sequential sonograms for 3-5 years are used to monitor

Prognosis
- Can be fatal when contralateral kidney is abnormal and oligohydramnios
- If contralateral kidney has delayed diagnosis of UPJ obstruction, renal insufficiency can be a problem
- Excellent when unilateral and uncomplicated
- Still excellent even when surgery required

Selected References
1.   Anderson et al: Detection of obstructive uropathy in the fetus. AJR 164:719-23, 1995
2.   Strife JL et al: Muticystic dysplastic kidney in children: US follow up. Radiology 186:785-8, 1993
3.   Reuss A et al: Sonographic, clinical and genetic aspects of prenatal diagnosis of cystic kidney disease. Ultrasound in Med & Biol 17:687-94, 1991

Ureteropelvic Junction Obstruction

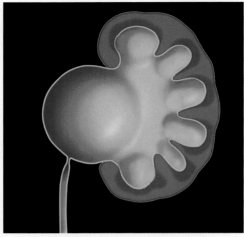

Drawing of ureteropelvic junction obstruction. Note proximal ureter is not dilated.

Key Facts
- Definition: Variable degree of obstruction to urine flow at the level of ureteropelvic junction (UPJ)
- Classic ultrasound appearance: Marked hydronephrosis that ends abruptly at the UPJ
- Obstruction is most often partial
- Most are nonprogressive in utero
- Follow-up studies needed to assess for change in severity of obstruction and postnatal studies needed to determine deterioration of renal function
- **Most common congenital malformation of the urinary tract**
- 30% are bilateral
- Oligohydramnios is rare
- Polyhydramnios may be paradoxically present
  - o Obstruction may impair kidney's ability to concentrate urine with subsequent high urine output

Imaging Findings
General Features
- Best imaging clue: Isolated hydronephrosis without ureteral or bladder dilatation
- Rarely may be complicated by a perirenal urinoma
Ultrasound Findings
- Moderate to severe hydronephrosis without hydroureter
- Fetal hydronephrosis: **Most sensitive criteria**
  - o AP diameter of renal pelvis
    - > or = 4 mm before 33 weeks
    - > or = 7 mm after 33 weeks
  - o Renal pelvis/kidney ratio > 0.28
  - o Calyceal dilatation
- Variable calyceal dilatation with or without renal cortical thinning
- Blunted or "bullet nosed" appearance at UPJ
- Fetal bladder is usually normal

Ureteropelvic Junction Obstruction

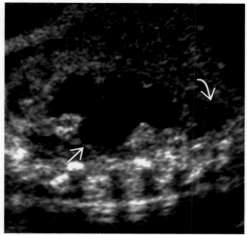

Ureteropelvic juction obstruction, second trimester fetus. Ultrasound shows the dilated pelvis and collecting system (arrow). Note the hypoechoic adrenal gland superior to the kidney (curved arrow).

- May initially look like a "cluster of cysts" but they connect with central large "cyst" (renal pelvis)

Imaging Recommendations
- When seen antenatally, follow up with ultrasound every 4-6 weeks
- **Wait at least 72 hours after delivery for postnatal ultrasound**
  - Dehydration minimizes hydronephrosis if done earlier

Differential Diagnosis

Hydronephrosis of Other Etiologies
- Vesicoureteral reflux
- UVJ obstruction
- Ureterocele
- Posterior urethral valves

Idiopathic Fetal Pyelectasis
- Seen in 2-3% of prenatal cases, may be related to maternal hydration
- Usually bilateral and never with calyceal distention

Fetal Pyelectasis Associated With Trisomy 21 (T21)
- Rarely an isolated finding, look for other markers for T21
- Isolated finding, increases risk 1.5 x baseline for that patient

Multicystic Dysplastic Kidney (MCDK)
- Cysts will not communicate

Pathology

General
- Theories of etiology of obstruction at the UPJ
  - Abnormal smooth muscle arrangement impairs distensibility
  - Abnormal innervation of proximal ureter – Hirschsprung's equivalent
  - Crossing vessel or fibrous scar at the UPJ
- Epidemiology
  - Most common congenital malformation of the urinary tract

Ureteropelvic Junction Obstruction

- Higher incidence of UPJ obstruction associated with MCDK
- These patients require prompt surgical intervention, since MCDK is nonfunctional and UPJ may compromise remaining renal function

Clinical Issues
Presentation
- Most often an incidental finding on prenatal sonogram
- Postnatally can become symptomatic with urinary tract infection, intermittent abdominal or flank pain, hematuria
- When seen on prenatal sonogram, need to assess kidneys postnatally
  - Wait at least 72 hours

Treatment
- In utero intervention or early delivery not usually indicated
- Postnatal
  - Pyeloplasty – open surgery resects narrowed segment at UPJ
  - Endoscopic incision - endopyelotomy
  - Percutaneous drainage as a temporizing measure, especially if infected

Prognosis
- Excellent if renal function has not been compromised by longstanding, high-grade obstruction
- Seen prenatally: Prognosis depends on opposite kidney appearance, amniotic fluid volume, presence of other anomalies
- Pelvicaliectasis persists for years on sonography following successful surgery – appropriate renal growth and good drainage on nuclear scans are measures of surgical success

Selected References
1. Kraus SJ: Genitourinary imaging in children. Pediatr Clin North Am 48:1381-424, 2001
2. Anderson N et al: Detection of obstructive uropathy in the fetus: Predictive value of sonographic measurements of renal pelvic diameter at various gestational ages. AJR 164:719-23, 1995
3. Corteville JE et al: Correlation of fetal ultrasonographic findings with infant outcome. Am J Obstet Gynecol 165:384-8,1991

Renal Duplication/Ureterocele

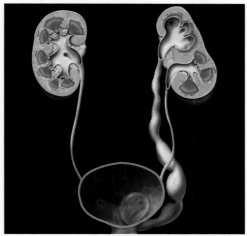

Renal duplication with ectopic ureterocele. Illustration shows a duplicated left-sided collecting system. The upper pole moiety is obstructed with ureteral dilatation and an ectopic ureterocele herniating into bladder lumen.

Key Facts
- Definition: Duplicated renal collecting system with prolapse of ectopic ureter into bladder
- Classic imaging appearance: Hydronephrosis involving upper pole with cystic mass in bladder
- Weigert-Meyer rule: Upper pole ureter inserts ectopically
  - Inferior and medial to normal ureter
    - **Upper pole obstructs**
    - **Lower pole refluxes**
- Bilateral 10-20%

Imaging Findings
General Features
- Best imaging clue: **Dilatation of upper pole collecting system with ureterocele** diagnostic
Ultrasound Findings
- Kidney
  - Dilatation of upper pole collecting system
    - May appear "cyst-like"
  - Reflux can intermittently dilate lower pole
  - Severe obstruction may result in dysplastic changes
- Ureter often dilated
- **Ectopic ureterocele**
  - Bladder most common insertion site
    - Less commonly urethra
    - Females: Vagina or uterus
    - Males: Seminal vesicles, ejaculatory ducts, vas deferens, epididymis
  - Thin-walled, "balloon-like" structure in bladder
    - Often large

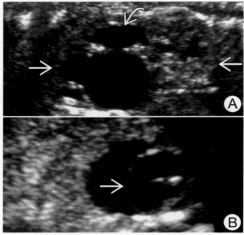

Renal duplication with ectopic ureterocele. (A) Longitudinal view of the left kidney (arrows) shows dilatation of the upper pole collecting system (curved arrow). (B) Transverse image of the bladder demonstrates a large ureterocele (arrow).

- May cause bladder outlet obstruction or obstruct contralateral kidney
  - Sagittal views may show direct connection with ureter
  - Color Doppler may show ureteral jet

Imaging Recommendations
- Evaluate kidney in both transverse and **longitudinal views**
  - Transverse views alone can lead to erroneous diagnosis of ureteropelvic junction (UPJ) obstruction
  - Lower pole moiety may be displaced inferiorly and difficult to see
  - Measure length
    - > 95% for gestational age
- Evaluate bladder several different times during study
  - **Ureterocele may be misinterpreted as bladder** if bladder is empty
  - Distended bladder may compress ureterocele
- Follow collecting system in real-time
  - Renal pelvis → ureter → ureterocele

Differential Diagnosis
UPJ Obstruction
- Entire collecting system dilated
- Ureter not seen
- No ureterocele

Reflux
- Entire collecting system dilated
- No ureterocele
- Findings may vary between scans

Simple Ureterocele
- Simple ureteroceles insert in normal location
- Not associated with renal duplication
- Not usually seen in utero

Renal Duplication/Ureterocele

Pathology

General

- General Path Comments
  - Renal duplication without ureterocele often missed
    - Look for band of parenchyma between upper and lower collecting system
    - Normal variant
- Genetics
  - Sporadic
- Etiology-Pathogenesis
  - Embryology
    - Accessory ureteric bud inserts separately into metanephric blastema
  - Orifice of ureterocele **stenotic** → ballooning of intravesicular segment
  - Ureterocele distorts adjacent normal ureteral orifice allowing **reflux**
- Epidemiology
  - Duplication with ectopic ureterocele
    - 1:9,000 live births
  - Duplication without ureterocele (ureters join before bladder insertion)
    - 1:150 in general population
    - No clinical significance

Clinical Issues

Presentation

- Incidental finding
- Evaluation of hydronephrosis

Treatment

- In utero treatment not usually indicated
- Complete workup after delivery
  - Voiding cystourethrogram (VCUG) for evaluating dynamic nature
    - Reflux, prolapse, obstruction
- Surgical options based on severity
  - Endoscopic incision
    - May convert obstructing ureterocele into refluxing one
  - Ureteral reimplantation
  - Heminephroureterectomy

Prognosis

- Excellent with early correction
- No recurrence risk

Selected References
1. Vergani P et al: Accuracy of prenatal ultrasonographic diagnosis of duplex renal system. J Ultrasound Med 18:463-7, 1999
2. Kang AH et al: Antenatal ultrasonographic development of ureteroceles. Implications for management. Fetal Diagn Ther 13:157-61, 1998
3. Abuhamad AZ et al: Renal duplication anomalies in the fetus: Clues for prenatal diagnosis. Ultrasound Obstet Gynecol 7:174-7, 1996

Posterior Urethral Valves

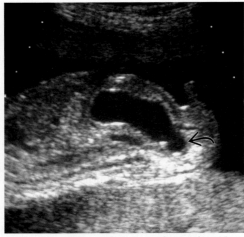

Posterior urethral valves. Midline sagittal view confirms male gender and shows an enlarged bladder with dilatation of the posterior urethra (arrow).

Key Facts
- Definition: Urethral membrane resulting in bladder outlet obstruction
- Classic imaging appearance: Distended bladder in a male fetus often with associated oligohydramnios
- High morbidity and mortality
  - Early diagnosis (< 24 weeks) & oligohydramnios poor prognostic signs
  - Fetal intervention may improve prognosis for select group
- **Cortical cysts best predictor for irreversible renal damage**
- Chromosomal abnormalities in 8-20%
- **Occurs exclusively in males**

Imaging Findings
General Features
- Best imaging clue: Distended bladder "funnels" into **dilated posterior urethra**
Ultrasound Findings
- Findings vary with degree of obstruction
- Bladder
  - Distended and thick-walled
    - May be huge and fill entire abdomen
  - **Dilated "keyhole" appearance of posterior urethra**
- Renal findings
  - Hydronephrosis
  - Ectatic ureters
  - **Renal dysplasia**
    - Echogenic kidneys
    - Small cortical cysts: Indicates irreversible damage
    - **Poor prognostic sign**
  - Perinephric urinoma
- Urinary ascites
  - Relieves pressure on kidneys

Posterior Urethral Valves

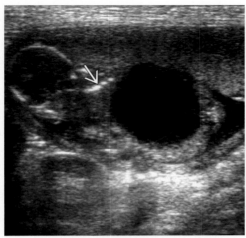

Posterior urethral valves. Grossly distended bladder in a 15 week fetus. Note the marked oligohydramnios and small, bell-shaped chest (arrow). Prognosis is dismal.

- o Favorable prognostic sign
- Oligohydramnios
  - o Small bell-shaped chest ⇒ pulmonary hypoplasia
- Associated malformations in 43%
  - o Cardiac malformations
  - o May be seen with VACTERL association

MR Findings
- Potential role in evaluating renal parenchyma for dysplastic changes

Imaging Recommendations
- Follow-up on all fetuses with large bladder
  - o Likely transient finding if otherwise normal appearance and fluid volume
- Evaluate for **poor prognostic signs**
  - o Echogenic kidneys (with or without cysts)
    - ▪ May precede abnormal urine chemistries
  - o Worsening bilateral hydronephrosis
    - ▪ Unilateral "protects" other kidney (better prognosis)
  - o Oligohydramnios

Differential Diagnosis

Urethral Atresia
- May have identical appearance
- Anhydramnios
- Male and female
- Much less common

Prune Belly Syndrome
- Lax or absent abdominal musculature
- Bladder thin-walled
- Entire urethra dilated
  - o Does not show characteristic "keyhole"

Posterior Urethral Valves

Megacystis Microcolon
- Bladder thin-walled
- No dilated posterior urethra
- **Fluid normal to increased**
- More common in females

Pathology
General
- Genetics: Sporadic
- Etiology-Pathogenesis
  - Abnormal thickening and/or fusion of normal circular mucosal folds
- Epidemiology
  - 1:8,000-25,000 live-born males
  - Higher incidence in utero
Gross Pathologic, Surgical Features
- Valve tissue is thin but forms a membrane obstructing antegrade flow

Clinical Issues
Presentation
- Oligohydramnios
- May be detected in 1st trimester
Treatment & Prognosis
- **Karyotype fetus** with either amniocentesis or bladder tap
- Termination offered
- > 32 wks worsening oligohydramnios ⇒ deliver ⇒ endoscopic valve ablation
- < 32 wks assess renal function
  - Perform serial bladder drainages over 3-4 days
  - Third sample most useful ("fresh" urine)
    - **Normal fetal urine is hypotonic**
  - Good prognostic indicators
    - Na < 100 mEq/L
    - Cl < 90 mEq/L
    - Osmolarity < 210 mOsm/L
    - β_2 microglobulin < 4 mg/L
    - Ca < 8 mg/dL
    - Sonographically normal kidneys (normal echogenicity, no cysts)
- Consider intervention for those in good prognostic category with worsening oligohydramnios and/or hydronephrosis
  - Vesicoamniotic shunt
    - Complications include shunt migration and occlusion
  - Vesicostomy if shunt fails
  - Experimental studies on in utero endoscopic valve ablation
- Overall mortality 25-50%
  - > 90% with oligohydramnios
- Up to half of survivors develop chronic renal insufficiency
- Long-term sequelae from poor bladder function

Selected References
1. Freedman AL et al: Fetal therapy for obstructive uropathy: Diagnosis specific outcomes [corrected]. J Urol 156:720-3; discussion 23-4, 1996
2. Crombleholme TM et al: Fetal intervention in obstructive uropathy: Prognostic indicators and efficacy of intervention. Am J Obstet Gynecol 162:1239-44, 1990
3. Mahony BS et al: Fetal renal dysplasia: Sonographic evaluation. Radiology 152:143-6, 1984

Mesoblastic Nephroma

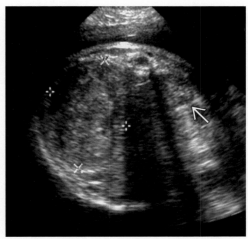

Mesoblastic nephroma. Axial sonogram of the fetal abdomen shows a large, solid mass within the right renal fossa (cursors). Note the normal-sized left kidney (arrow).

Key Facts

- Synonym: Leiomyomatous hamartoma, mesenchymal hamartoma
- Definition: Hamartomatous renal tumor composed predominately of spindle cells
  - Generally benign
  - Cellular variant potentially more aggressive
- Classic imaging appearance: A large, unilateral, predominately solid renal mass
- **Polyhydramnios** common feature and may be severe (etiology uncertain)
  - Some infants with mesoblastic nephroma have hypercalcemia which has been associated with polyuria
    - Potential explanation for increased amniotic fluid
- Rare but **most common in utero renal tumor**
  - Generally seen in 3rd trimester
- Most present in first 3 months of life

Imaging Findings

General Features

- Best imaging clue: No normal kidney visualized on side of mass
- Pertinent negatives
  - Hemorrhage or necrosis uncommon
  - Hydronephrosis not present

Ultrasound Findings

- Smaller masses retain reniform shape
  - Infiltrative growth pattern
- Larger masses may fill abdomen displacing bowel
  - Bowel obstruction may occur
- Variable echogenecity
- Vascular on color Doppler

Mesoblastic Nephroma

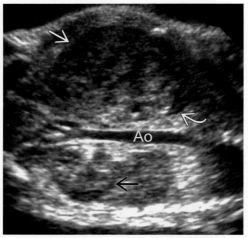

Mesoblastic nephroma. Coronal sonogram in the same fetus shows a markedly enlarged right kidney (white arrow). Compare to the normal-sized left kidney (black arrow). Note the normal adrenal gland is seen above the renal mass (curved arrow). (Ao - aorta).

MR Findings
- Helpful to confirm if mass is renal

Imaging Recommendations
- Identify normal adrenal gland to confirm mass is renal
- Frequent follow-up exams for
  - Worsening polyhydramnios
    - May become severe resulting in preterm labor
  - Enlarging abdominal circumference
  - Rarely complicated by hydrops

Differential Diagnosis

Neuroblastoma
- **Suprarenal location**
- Kidney displaced inferiorly
- Normal adrenal gland not identified

Adrenal Hemorrhage
- Will evolve over time
- No color flow within mass
- MRI can confirm blood products

Wilms Tumor
- Ultrasound appearance identical
- Extraordinarily rare in utero
  - Average age at presentation 3.6 years

Autosommal Recessive Polycystic Kidney Disease
- Bilateral enlargement

Multicystic Dysplastic Kidney
- Cystic not solid

Mesoblastic Nephroma

Pathology

<u>General</u>
- Genetics
  - Sporadic
  - No recurrence risk
- Epidemiology
  - Rare
  - M > F

<u>Gross Pathologic, Surgical Features</u>
- Whorled appearance
  - Similar to uterine fibroid
- No capsule
  - Still appears well defined by ultrasound

Clinical Issues

<u>Presentation</u>
- Polyhydramnios
  - Large for dates
  - Preterm labor

<u>Natural History</u>
- Can show rapid growth despite benign histology
- Large abdominal circumference may result in dystocia at delivery

<u>Treatment</u>
- Amnioreduction for polyhydramnios
- Tocolytics for preterm labor
- Referral to pediatric urologist
- Resection in neonatal period
  - **Nephrectomy** with wide margins usually curative

<u>Prognosis</u>
- Excellent
  - Chemotherapy or radiation not usually indicated
- Rare local recurrence or metastases
  - Lung most common site

Selected References
1. Irsutti M et al: Mesoblastic nephroma: Prenatal ultrasonographic and MRI features. Pediatr Radiol 30:147-50, 2000
2. Fung TY et al: Polyhydramnios and hypercalcemia associated with congenital mesoblastic nephroma: Case report and a new appraisal. Obstet Gynecol 85:815-7, 1995
3. Walter JP et al: Mesoblastic nephroma: Prenatal sonographic detection. J Clin Ultrasound 13:686-9, 1985

Neuroblastoma

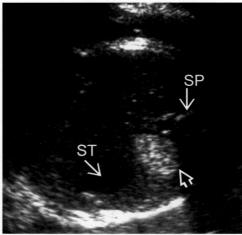

Neuroblastoma in a 30 week fetus. Transverse sonogram of the fetal abdomen shows a well-defined, echogenic mass (open arrow) posterior to the stomach (ST) and adjacent to the spine (SP). This appearance is identical to that of an extralobar sequestration but no feeding vessel was identified on color Doppler.

Key Facts
- Definition: Malignant tumor composed of neuroblasts arising within sympathetic neural plexus or adrenal medulla
- Classic imaging appearance: **Solid and/or cystic suprarenal retroperitoneal mass**
- **> 90% adrenal** origin
  - Differs from neonatal period when only 45% are adrenal
- Presents in 3rd trimester
- Elevated catecholamines may cause symptoms in mother
  - Preeclampsia, headaches, tachycardia
  - Indicates advanced stage disease
- Majority have **favorable stage (1, 2, or 4-S) and biologic markers**
- **Amniocentesis** may help in diagnosis
  - Elevated catecholamines in amniotic fluid reported

Imaging Findings
<u>General Features</u>
- Best imaging clue: No identifiable adrenal gland on side of mass
<u>Ultrasound Findings</u>
- Variable echogenicity
  - Uniformly echogenic
  - Approximately **half are cystic**
  - Rarely calcified
    - Less common than pediatric age group
- Color Doppler shows flow in mass
  - Does not have single feeding vessel
- Hepatic metastases may be difficult to identify
<u>MR Findings</u>
- Useful for staging and evaluating metastases
- Can accurately exclude adrenal hemorrhage from differential

Neuroblastoma

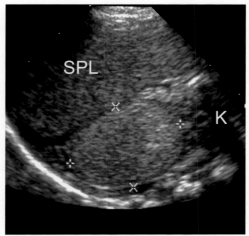

Neuroblastoma. Longitudinal sonogram of the same infant after delivery shows an echogenic mass (cursors) superior to the kidney (K). Diagnosis was confirmed at surgery. (SPL - spleen).

Imaging Recommendations
- Careful examination for metastases
  - Liver
  - Placenta (rare)
    - Microscopic tumor emboli
    - Bulky, hydropic placenta
    - Discrete masses less likely
- Consider MRI if mother has preeclampsia
  - Suggests advanced disease
  - Look for metastases
- Follow for growth and developing hydrops

Differential Diagnosis
Extralobar Sequestion
- **More likely** than neuroblastoma as cause of left-sided suprarenal mass
  - 10% are below diaphragm
  - Usually on left
  - Presents earlier
- **Dominant feeding vessel from aorta**
- Uniformly echogenic
- Separate adrenal gland may be identified
Adrenal Hemorrhage
- Will evolve over time
- No color flow within mass
- MRI can confirm blood products
Mesoblastic Nephroma
- Renal mass
- Adrenal gland is normal

Neuroblastoma

Pathology
General
- Genetics
  - Rare familial cases
- Favorable DNA index
- Absent Myc-N amplification
  - Proto-oncogene on chromosome 2p
    - Multiple copies (>10) in aggressive tumors

Staging Criteria
- 1: Confined to organ of interest
- 2: Extension beyond organ but not crossing midline
- 3: Extension crossing midline
- 4: Distant metastases
- **4S: Metastatic disease confined to skin, liver, and bone marrow, age < 1 year**
  - Near 100% survival

Clinical Issues
Presentation
- Generally incidental finding in **3rd trimester**
  - Adrenal most common
  - Thoracic and cervical masses reported
- Rarely preeclampsia or headaches

Natural History
- Variable course
  - **May resolve spontaneously**
  - Most remain stable without complications
    - Tumors may "mature" to more benign histologic type (ganglioneuroblastoma and ganglioneuroma)
  - A minority progress to hydrops and even death

Treatment
- Consider early delivery if rapidly growing or metastases detected
- Surgical resection after delivery
  - Chemotherapy or radiation not usually indicated
- No treatment advocated by some for favorable stage disease

Prognosis
- > 90% survival overall
- Poor for stages 3 and 4

Selected References
1. Lonergan GJ et al: Neuroblastoma, ganglioneuroblastoma, and ganglioneuroma: radiologic-pathologic correlation. Radiographics 22:911-34, 2002
2. Acharya S et al: Prenatally diagnosed neuroblastoma. Cancer 80:304-10, 1997
3. Curtis MR et al: Prenatal ultrasound characterization of the suprarenal mass: distinction between neuroblastoma and subdiaphragmatic extralobar pulmonary sequestration. J Ultrasound Med 16:75-83, 1997

Ovarian Cyst

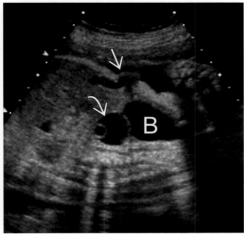

Ovarian cyst. Midline sagittal image of the abdomen in a 3ʳᵈ trimester female fetus shows a cyst superior to the bladder (curved arrow). It is slightly complex with a smaller cyst within it. (B - bladder, arrow - cord insertion).

Key Facts
- Definition: Benign functional cyst within fetal ovary
- Classic imaging appearance: Anechoic abdominal cyst in female fetus
- **Most common cause** of abdominal cyst in a 3ʳᵈ trimester female fetus
  - Do not consider in differential for cysts diagnosed earlier in pregnancy
- Results from excessive maternal and placental hormones
- Can be **located anywhere in abdomen**
  - Supporting ligaments are lax

Imaging Findings
General Features
- Best imaging clue: Abdominal cyst in **3ʳᵈ trimester** female fetus
- Vary in size but may be large (up to 10 cm)
  - Can cause bowel obstruction
    - Polyhydramnios may develop
- Most unilateral but occasionally bilateral
- Ascites if cyst ruptures

Ultrasound Findings
- Generally anechoic and unilocular
  - May have occasional septations
- Internal echoes indicate hemorrhage usually from torsion
  - Variable appearance based on age
    - Diffusely echogenic
    - Fluid/fluid level
    - Crescentic or rounded as clot retracts
  - Doppler not often helpful

Imaging Recommendations
- Confirm cyst is intraperitoneal and separate from urinary tract
  - **Most cystic abdominal masses are related to urinary tract**
- Document sex

Ovarian Cyst

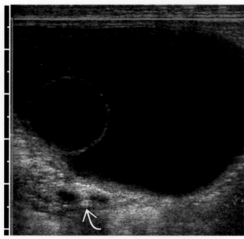

Ovarian cyst. Linear sonographic image on day 1 of life in the same case shows the cyst to be predominately anechoic with a smaller cyst within it. A crescent of normal parenchyma with two small cysts is seen confirming it is ovarian in origin (curved arrow). The cyst resolved on follow-up exams.

Differential Diagnosis

Urachal Cyst
- Between dome of bladder and cord insertion
- Occurs in both males and females

Hydrocolpos
- Midline pelvic mass
- Posterior to bladder

Duplication Cyst
- Presents earlier in 2nd trimester
- Occurs in both males and females
- May appear identical

Mesenteric Cyst
- Occurs in both males and females
- May appear identical
- Much less common

Choledochal Cyst
- Right upper quadrant
- Associated with liver

Dilated Bowel
- Tubular configuration
- Contents echogenic (succus entericus)
- Peristalsis confirmatory

Meconium Pseudocyst
- Often irregular contour
- Wall can calcify
- Other sequelae of meconium peritonitis
  - Peritoneal calcifications
  - Dilated bowel

Ovarian Cyst

Pathology

General

- Etiology-Pathogenesis
  - o Response to increased hormone levels
  - o Associated with fetal hypothyroidism
- Epidemiology
  - o 1/3 of infant girls have cysts
    - ▪ Most microscopic
    - ▪ Rare to be large enough for US detection

Clinical Issues

Presentation

- Usually incidental finding in 3rd trimester

Natural History

- Rarely complicated by hemorrhage or torsion
  - o Risk increases with cyst size
- Most show substantial regression by 6 months of age
  - o May take up to 2 years for complete resolution

Treatment

- Prenatal cyst drainage
  - o Usually only done for large cysts with bowel obstruction or at risk for dystocia
  - o Some advocate for cysts > 4 cm to prevent torsion
  - o Elevated progesterone and estradiol in cyst fluid is diagnostic
- US after delivery to confirm ovarian location
- Follow monthly until resolved
- Indications for surgical resection
  - o Evidence of torsion
  - o Bowel or urinary tract obstruction
  - o Failure to resolve
    - ▪ Controversial as all will eventually resolve
    - ▪ No malignant potential
- **Surgery should preserve ovarian parenchyma**

Prognosis

- Excellent if no torsion

Selected References
1.   Crombleholme TM et al: Fetal ovarian cyst decompression to prevent torsion. J Pediatr Surg 32:1447-9, 1997
2.   Muller-Leisse C et al: Ovarian cysts in the fetus and neonate-changes in sonographic pattern in the follow-up and their management. Pediatr Radiol 22:395-400, 1992
3.   Meizner I et al: Fetal ovarian cysts: Prenatal ultrasonographic detection and postnatal evaluation and treatment. Am J Obstet Gynecol 164:874-8, 1991

Sacrococcygeal Teratoma

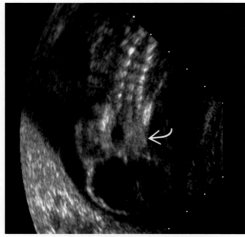

Sacrococcygeal teratoma. Ultrasound image shows cystic mass extending from fetal perineum. Possible solid components seen on ultrasound (curved arrow). Note apparent widening interpedicular distance causing confusion with myelomeningocele. Serial transverse images showed spine was normal.

Key Facts

- Definition: Neoplasm derived from all three germ cell layers
- Classic imaging appearance: Exophytic mass extending from fetal sacrum
- Fetal tumors generally benign
- **Hypervascular**: Risk high output cardiac failure/hemorrhage
- Can be large
  - o Obstructed labor: Dystocia 6-13%
  - o Intrapartum trauma: Risk fetal exsanguination
- Some cases may benefit from fetal surgery

Imaging Findings

<u>General Features</u>
- Best imaging clue: Exophytic mixed cystic/solid mass extending from sacrum
- Anatomy: American Academy of Pediatrics Surgery Section (AAPSS)
  - o Type 1: Completely external or minimal presacral component
  - o Type 2: External and internal component extending into pelvis
  - o Type 3: External and internal component extending into abdomen
  - o Type 4: Completely internal, no external component
    - ▪ Most likely to undergo malignant degeneration (postnatal)
    - ▪ Malignancy more likely in solid than cystic or mixed

<u>Ultrasound Findings</u>
- Mixed solid/cystic mass
  - o Purely cystic forms have been reported
  - o May contain calcifications
- Placentomegaly
- Polyhydramnios ⇒ increased risk preterm labor
- Color Doppler demonstrates vascularity

Sacrococcygeal Teratoma

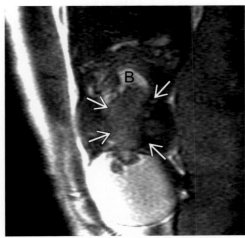

Sacrococcygeal teratoma. Coronal SSFSE image from fetal MRI on the same patient shows significant internal soft tissue component (arrows) displacing bladder (B) superiorly. This fetus was delivered by C-section and had uncomplicated single stage excision of the mass.

MR Findings
- SSFSE
  - Exquisite demonstration internal component
  - Low signal blood products within mass confirm hemorrhage
- FMPSPGR
  - Blood products high signal: **Will differentiate enlargement due to bleed from rapid growth**
  - Fatty components high signal both sequences

Imaging Recommendations
- Echocardiography for high output state
  - Very poor prognosis if hydrops develops
- Track size of lesion: Volume cystic/solid components
  - Unpredictable growth
  - Reports of mass reaching 25 cm diameter
- Careful search for associated malformations: 11-38%
  - Mostly local secondary to tumor growth
    - Imperforate anus
    - Obstructive uropathy

Differential Diagnosis
Myelomeningocele (MMC)
- Spinal defect present
- Contains neural elements
- Almost all MMC associated with Chiari II malformation
  - "Lemon" sign of frontal concavity: Invariably resolved by 34 weeks
  - "Banana" sign of cerebellum with obliterated cisterna magna
- Beware: **MMC and Sacrococcygeal Teratoma (SCGT) may occur together**

Sacrococcygeal Teratoma

<u>Other Solid Tumors</u>
- > 50 masses/malformations described in sacrococcygeal area
- All rarer that SCGT

Pathology
<u>General</u>
- Genetics: No reported cases with aneuploidy
- Etiology-Pathogenesis
  - Embryology
    - Remnants of primitive streak
    - Pluripotent cells
    - Tumor contains all 3 germ layers
    - Incomplete differentiation
- Epidemiology
  - 1:35,000
  - Commonest neonatal tumor
  - M:F = 1:4
  - Malignant change M > F

Clinical Issues
<u>Presentation</u>
- Described as early as 13.5 weeks
- Often presents as size > dates
  - Large mass
  - Polyhydramnios
<u>Treatment</u>
- Monitor mother for preeclampsia/"mirror" syndrome
- Scan weekly for size of mass and signs hydrops
- Deliver in tertiary center at lung maturity
- C-section preferred if tumor > 5 cm
  - Larger masses may require classical incision
  - Aspiration of cystic lesions may allow vaginal delivery
- Fetal surgery
  - Must have normal karyotype
  - Predominantly solid: Increased risk hydrops independent of tumor size
  - Limited experience but "viable option"
<u>Prognosis</u>
- Fetal diagnosis: 50% mortality related to high output state
  - Newborn diagnosis: ≤ 5% mortality related to malignancy
- Worse outcome if
  - Maternal indication for scan e.g., large for dates
  - Diagnosed at < 30 weeks
  - Hydrops ⇒ almost always fatal
- Better outcome if cystic
  - Less vascular ⇒ decreased risk hemorrhage, hydrops

Selected References
1. Avni FE et al: MR imaging of fetal sacrococcygeal teratoma. AJR 178:179-83, 2002
2. Coleman B et al: Fetal therapy: State of the Art. J Ultrasound Med 21:1257-88, 2002
3. Altman RP et al: Sacrococcygeal teratoma: American Academy of Pediatrics Surgical Section survey-1973. J Pediatr Surg 9:389-98, 1974

PocketRadiologist®
Obstetrics
Top 100 Diagnoses

SKELETAL

Achondroplasia

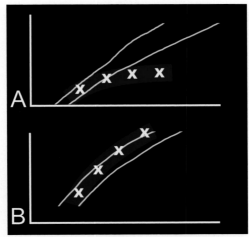

Achondroplasia. (A) Femur length. On the initial scan the femur length is normal. A decrease in interval growth is noted in mid-pregnancy with obvious shortening in the 3rd trimester. (B) Head circumference plot shows an enlarged head.

Key Facts
- Definition: Rhizomelic skeletal dysplasia occurring in 2 forms
  - Heterozygous: **Most common nonlethal skeletal dysplasia**
  - Homozygous: Lethal
- Classic imaging appearance: Marked shortening of long bones with large head and frontal bossing
- Single gene defect on chromosome 4p
- **Cannot be diagnosed before 22 weeks**
  - Homozygous may be detected earlier
- Autosomal dominant disorder but 80% new mutations

Imaging Findings
General Features
- Best imaging clue: Normal early scan with long bone shortening noted after 22 weeks
- Rhizomelic dysplasia: Proximal limb shortening
Ultrasound Findings
- **Ossification is normal**
- No bowing or angulation
- **Large head with frontal bossing**
- Flat, **depressed nasal bridge**
- Chest normal to mildly narrowed
- **Trident hands**
  - Fingers all same length
  - **3rd and 4th fingers gapped**
- Bone growth
  - Manifests between 21-27 weeks
  - Progressive discrepant growth
    - Shortening more obvious in 3rd trimester

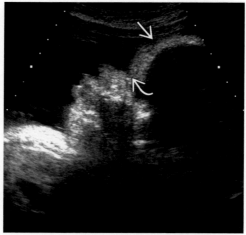

Achondroplasia. Profile view of a fetus with achondroplasia. Note the frontal bossing (arrow) and depressed nasal bridge (curved arrow).

- Head circumference (HC)/femur length (FL) increases (function of both short femur and large head)
  - o Upper extremities more severely affected
- Polyhydramnios may develop in 3rd trimester
- Decreased interpedicular distance in lumbar spine
- 3D ultrasound useful for evaluating hands and spine
- **Homozygous form**
  - o Findings more severe and seen earlier
  - o At risk patients (one or both affected parents) should have serial sonograms for growth
    - FL < 3% at 17 weeks
    - FL < 34 mm at 26 weeks by biparietal diameter (BPD)

Radiographic Findings
- Radiographs may be taken in 3rd trimester to better evaluate bone morphology and ossification
  - o Positioning under fluoroscopy with spot films preferred to KUB
    - Fetal bones often overlap maternal spine

Imaging Recommendations
- Follow-up sonogram if femur lagging behind other measurements
  - o **Heterozygous form becomes obvious in 3rd trimester**
- Rule out lethal dysplasia
  - o Micromelia
  - o Small chest

Differential Diagnosis
Osteogenesis Imperfecta
- Fractures dominant feature
- Decreased ossification
Spondyloepiphyseal Dysplasia
- Rhizomelic dysplasia with similar long bone features
- No frontal bossing

- Micrognathia may be present

Thanatophoric Dysplasia
- More severe shortening (micromelia)
- Small chest
- Curved long bones
- "Cloverleaf" skull

Pathology

General
- General Path Comments
  - Hypochondroplasia milder form of achondroplasia
    - Not usually detected in utero
  - No increased incidence of major organ anomalies
- Genetics
  - Autosomal dominant
  - **Homozygous achondroplasia is lethal**
  - **80% of cases are new mutations**
- Etiology-Pathogenesis
  - Decreased endochondral ossification
  - Defect on chromosome 4p
    - Mutation of the fibroblast growth factor receptor - 3 (**FGFR3**)
  - Associated with **advanced paternal age**
- Epidemiology
  - Heterozygous: 1:10,000-30,000 live births
  - Homozygous: rare
    - Both parents must be affected or one parent + new mutation

Clinical Issues

Presentation
- Long bone shortening in late 2nd and 3rd trimester

Treatment
- Patients should undergo genetic counseling
- FGFR-3 mutation can be diagnosed by amniocentesis or chorionic villus sampling

Prognosis
- Generally normal lifespan and intelligence
- Increased incidence of orthopedic and neurologic complications
  - Cervical instability
  - Spinal stenosis
  - Limb bowing
- One affected parent recurrence risk 25%
- Two affected parents recurrence risk 50%
  - 25% risk of homozygous form
- New mutation no increased risk

Selected References
1. Patel MD et al: Homozygous achondroplasia: US distinction between homozygous, heterozygous, and unaffected fetuses in the second trimester. Radiology 196:541-5, 1995
2. Guzman ER et al: Prenatal ultrasonographic demonstration of the trident hand in heterozygous achondroplasia. J Ultrasound Med 13:63-6, 1994
3. Kurtz AB et al: In utero analysis of heterozygous achondroplasia: Variable time of onset as detected by femur length measurements. J Ultrasound Med 5:137-40, 1986

Achondrogenesis

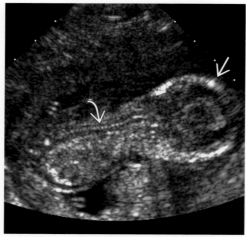

Achondrogenesis Type 2. Coronal sonogram of the fetus shows a relatively large head in relation to the torso. Note the normal skull ossification (arrow). There is almost absent mineralization of the spine (curved arrow). There was also marked shortening of the lower extremities with no normally ossified long bones.

Key Facts
- Synonym: Chondrogenesis imperfecta
- Definition: Lethal skeletal dysplasia due to failure of cartilaginous matrix formation
- Classic imaging appearance
  - Severe micromelia
  - Markedly decreased bone mineralization
- Type 1 (Parenti-Fraccaro)
  - Severe limb shortening
  - Generalized poor ossification
  - Minimal spine ossification
  - Rib fractures
- Type 2 (Langer-Saldino)
  - Limb shortening variable
  - Relatively normal skull ossification
  - **Complete lack ossification spine/pelvis**

Imaging Findings
General Features
- Best imaging clue: Type 1
  - Generalized deficient mineralization
  - Rib fractures
    - Fractures **not** predominant feature
- Best imaging clue: Type 2
  - Normal skull ossification
  - Absent spine mineralization
    - Uniformly hypoechoic
    - No visible ossification centers

Achondrogenesis

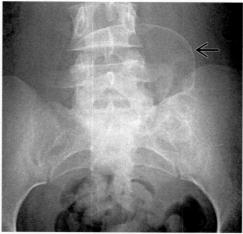

Achondrogenesis Type 2. Fetal skeletal survey at 30 weeks gestation. Only the skull vault (arrow) is ossified hence the term "floating head."

Ultrasound Findings
- Short flared ribs
- Micrognathia
- Large head size
- Short trunk
- Hydrops
- Polyhydramnios
- Increased nuchal lucency/cystic hygroma
- Skin thickening

Fetal Skeletal Survey Findings
- Type 2: "Floating head"
  - Only skull ossified well enough to be seen
  - Normal clavicles

Imaging Recommendations
- Attempt to measure all long bones
- Facial images
  - Micrognathia
  - Cleft palate

Differential Diagnosis

Osteogenesis Imperfecta (OI)
- Fractures are **predominant** finding in OI
  - Rib fractures occur in Type 1 achondrogenesis
    - **Not** dominant feature
  - Fractures **not** seen in Type 2 achondrogenesis
- Skull poorly mineralized in OI

Hypophosphatasia
- Skull demineralized
- Multiple long-bone **fractures**

Achondrogenesis

Atelosteogenesis
- **Thoracic platyspondyly**
- Bowed radius, ulna, tibia
- Clubfeet

Pathology
General
- General Path Comments
  - Cartilaginous matrix does not form
  - No matrix = no bone
- Genetics
  - Type 1: Autosomal recessive
    - 25% recurrence risk
  - Type 2: Sporadic
    - Negligible recurrence risk
    - Mutation of COL2A1 gene
- Epidemiology
  - Rare sporadic incidence
  - Reported cases show excess of males
  - Can be diagnosed as early as 12 to 14 weeks

Clinical Issues
Natural History
- Lethal
Treatment
- Offer termination
- If pregnancy progresses and diagnosis certain
  - Avoid fetal monitoring in labor
  - Allow pre-term labor to proceed
  - Psychological support for family
- If diagnosis unclear and live born infant, resuscitation appropriate until confirmatory tests performed
- Stress importance of full genetic evaluation
- Autopsy important for final specific diagnosis
  - X-rays
    - Absent mineralization of spine
  - Cell culture
  - Bone/cartilage biopsy
- Deliver in tertiary center with expertise in fetal pathology/skeletal dysplasia
Prognosis
- Lethal
- Recurrence risk depends on type

Selected References
1. Korkko J et al: Widely distributed mutations in the COL2A1 gene produce achondrogenesis type II/hypochondrogenesis. Am J Med Genet 92:95-100, 2000
2. Jaeger H et al: The boneless neonate: A severe form of achondrogenesis type 1. Pediatr Radiol 24:319-21, 1994
3. Anteby S et al: Prenatal diagnosis of achondrogenesis. Radiol Clin (Basel) 46:109-14, 1977

Thanatophoric Dysplasia

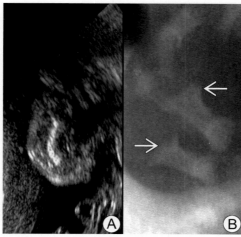

Thanatophoric dysplasia. Ultrasound image (A) of the lower extremity shows curved femur. Femur length more than two standard deviations below mean for GA. Fetal skeletal survey (B) at 30 weeks gestation shows short femurs with marked metaphyseal flaring (arrows).

Key Facts
- Synonyms: TD, fatal skeletal dysplasia, thanatophoric dwarfism
- Definition: Lethal skeletal dysplasia due to mutation of fibroblast growth factor 3 gene
- Classic imaging appearance
  - Short limbed dwarfism: May be rhizomelic
  - Bowed long bones
  - Platyspondyly
  - Small chest
  - Protuberant abdomen
  - Trident hand
  - Hydrocephalus
  - Redundant skin
- Most common lethal skeletal dysplasia
  - **Any severe micromelia carries poor prognosis**
  - Exact prenatal diagnosis can be challenging
  - Exact diagnosis will not impact pregnancy management but will impact counseling on recurrence risk

Imaging Findings
Ultrasound Findings
- Best imaging clue
  - "Telephone receiver" femur classic for TD type 1
  - Kleeblattschadel (cloverleaf) skull classic for TD type 2
- Type 1
  - Relatively normal skull
  - Long bones, < 5% for GA
  - **Curved long bones** especially "telephone receiver" femur
  - Small thorax, short ribs
  - Depressed bridge of nose, frontal bossing

Thanatophoric Dysplasia

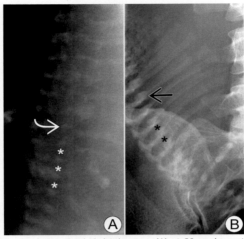

Thanatophoric dysplasia. Fetal skeletal survey (A) at 30 weeks gestation shows severe platyspondyly (curved arrow). The disc height (*) is greater than the vertebral body height. Incidental fetal spine image (B) in pregnant trauma patient shows normal vertebral bodies (arrow) and disc heights (*).

- Type 2
  - **Cloverleaf** (Kleeblattschadel) skull
  - Femurs less curved
  - Platyspondyly less marked
- 75% severe polyhydramnios by late 2nd trimester

Fetal Skeletal Survey
- Platyspondyly: Better seen than on US
- Flared irregular metaphyses

Imaging Recommendations
- Measure all long bones
- Fetal skeletal survey in 3rd trimester
- 3D US useful for spatial relationships
  - Absent bones
  - Scapular hypoplasia/aplasia
  - Short ribs
  - Splayed digits

Differential Diagnosis

Achondrogenesis
- Absent spine ossification
  - Spine ossification present in TD

Homozygous Achondroplasia
- Look at parents!
- May not be apparent until > 20 weeks

Camptomelic Dysplasia
- Hypoplastic scapula
- Hypoplastic fibulae
- Upper extremities < lower
- Sharp **bowing angulation** femur and tibia

Thanatophoric Dysplasia

Pathology

General

- General Path Comments
  - Femoral growth zones show abnormal ossification
  - Temporal lobe heterotopias
  - Other microscopic abnormalities in CNS
- Genetics
  - Sporadic new dominant mutation of FGFR3 gene
- Etiology-Pathogenesis
  - FGFR3 member of tyrosine kinase receptor family
  - Tyrosine kinase important in cell growth and differentiation
  - Ultimately abnormal chondrocyte differentiation
- Epidemiology
  - 1:10-40,000 live births in USA
  - M=F

Clinical Issues

Presentation

- Can be detected by 14 weeks

Natural History

- Lethal within first few days of life
  - Small thorax: Pulmonary hypoplasia
  - Abnormal skull/spine/small foramen magnum: Brainstem compression

Treatment

- Amniocentesis
  - Molecular testing for FGFR3 gene mutations
- Offer termination
- If pregnancy progresses and diagnosis certain
  - Avoid fetal monitoring in labor
  - Allow pre-term labor to proceed
  - Psychological support for family
- If diagnosis unclear and infant liveborn, resuscitation appropriate until confirmatory tests performed
- **Autopsy important for final specific diagnosis**
  - X-rays **even if** prenatal survey performed
  - Bone/cartilage biopsy
- Deliver in tertiary center with expertise in fetal pathology/skeletal dysplasia

Prognosis

- No significant recurrence risk

Selected References
1. Chen CP et al: Second trimester molecular diagnosis of a stop codon FGF3 mutation in a type 1 thanatophoric dysplasia fetus following abnormal ultrasound findings. Prenat Diagnosis 22:736-7, 2002
2. Kolbe N et al: Diagnosis of skeletal dysplasia by multidisciplinary assessment: A report of two cases of thanatophoric dysplasia. Ultrasound Obstet Gynecol 19:92-8, 2002
3. Garjian K et al: Fetal skeletal dysplasia: Three-dimensional US-initial experience. Radiology 214:717-23, 2000

Osteogenesis Imperfecta

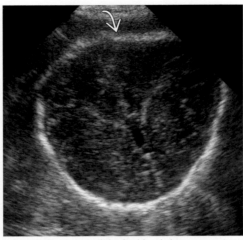

Osteogenesis imperfecta. Image of the fetal head shows poor mineralization with very little shadowing from the skull. Also note the transducer is flattening and deforming the skull (arrow).

Key Facts
- Definition: Skeletal dysplasia characterized by increased propensity to fracture
- Classic imaging appearance: **Multiple long bone and rib fractures**
- Osteogenesis imperfecta (OI) occurs in 4 types
  - Type II most common type diagnosed in utero
    - Lethal in neonatal period

Imaging Findings
General Features
- Best imaging clue: Presence of fractures distinguishes OI from other skeletal dysplasias
- **Classification System:** Based on phenotype
  - Type I: Limb abnormalities develop after birth
  - Type II: Most severe form, multiple fractures
    - Small chest
    - Severe limb shortening
    - Demineralization of skull
  - Type III: Multiple fractures at birth
    - Progressive deformity
    - Detectable by 2nd trimester
  - Type IV: Delayed presentation
    - Early onset osteoporosis 4th to 5th decades

Ultrasound Findings
- **Normal ultrasound does not exclude OI in high-risk patient**
- Extremities
  - Long bone shortening secondary to fractures
  - Angulation
  - Callous formation
    - May give bone an irregular "bumpy" appearance

Osteogenesis Imperfecta

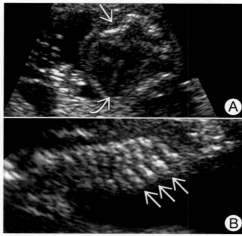

Osteogenesis imperfecta. (A) Axial image at the level of the heart (curved arrow) shows a small chest with concave, irregular ribs (arrow). (B) In the sagittal plane the ribs have a wavy, beaded, irregular appearance (arrows).

- o Decreased mineralization
  - ▪ May see posterior cortex (i.e., no shadowing from anterior cortex)
  - ▪ Bones appear "thick" but short
- Chest
  - o Small chest
  - o Short concave ribs
  - o Multiple fractures ⇒ "beading"
- Brain
  - o Anatomy "too well seen"
    - ▪ Poorly mineralized skull
    - ▪ No reverberation artifact
  - o Transducer pressure may deform skull

Radiographic Findings
- Fractures may be better demonstrated on fetal skeletal survey

Imaging Recommendations
- Measure all long bones
  - o Severe rhizomelia
- Look for scapulae
  - o If visible camptomelic dysplasia unlikely
- Compare chest to abdominal circumference
  - o Small chest ⇒ more risk for respiratory compromise at birth
- Monitor fluid volume
  - o Associated with polyhydramnios
- Watch for hydrocephalus
  - o Head size may impact delivery plan

Differential Diagnosis

Hypophosphatasia
- No fractures

Osteogenesis Imperfecta

Achondrogenesis (AG)
- Spine mineralization absent in AG type II

Camptomelic Dysplasia
- Hypoplastic scapulae
- Sharp angled bowing of tibia/femur

Pathology

General
- Genetics
  - Most autosomal dominant
  - Autosomal recessive inheritance described especially with type II
  - Mosaicism and new mutations common
  - COL1A1, COL1A2 genes control type 1 collagen production
- Etiology-Pathogenesis
  - Abnormal type 1 collagen
  - Decreased bone mineralization
  - Increased bone fragility
- Epidemiology
  - 4:100,000 live births (50% Type 2)

Gross Pathologic, Surgical Features
- OI Type II
  - Thin cortical bone, sparse trabecular bone
  - Increased osteoclasts/osteocytes
  - Thin osteoid with thin collagen fibrils
  - Patchy mineralization

Clinical Issues

Presentation
- Detected as early as 13-14 weeks
- May have family history

Treatment
- Genetic counseling
- Biochemical and collagen analysis from CVS or amniocentesis
  - Must know precise defect in the family
  - Cultivate fibroblasts or amniocytes
    - May take 30 days to grow
  - Significant collagen in chorionic villi
    - Direct extraction $\Rightarrow$ results 3-5 days
- Cesarean section for non-lethal forms
  - Less chance of birth trauma
- Encourage autopsy if termination/demise
  - Culture cell line for precise biochemical defect

Prognosis
- Variable according to type
- Neonatal demise common in type II
  - Rib fractures $\Rightarrow$ small chest $\Rightarrow$ pulmonary compromise

Selected References
1. Ries L et al: Prenatal diagnosis of a novel COL1A1 mutation in osteogenesis imperfecta type 1 carried through full term pregnancy. Prenat Diagn 20:876-80, 2000
2. Sarathchandra P et al: A light and electron microscope study of osteogenesis imperfecta bone samples, with reference to collagen chemistry and clinical phenotype. J Pathol 192:385 95, 2000
3. Raghunath M et al: Prenatal diagnosis of collagen disorders by direct biochemical analysis of chorionic villus biopsies. Pediatr Res 36:441-8, 1994

Arthrogryposis

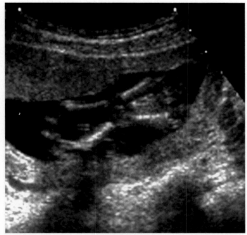

Arthrogryposis. Ultrasound image shows abnormal positioning with fixed extension of the lower extremities. The fetus had multiple congenital anomalies and maternal serum screening showed elevated risk for trisomy 18.

Key Facts
- Synonyms: Fetal hypokinesia/akinesia sequence, multiple congenital contractures, Pena Shokeir **phenotype** (catch all expression for this physical appearance)
- Definition: Multiple congenital joint contractures involving **two or more body areas**
- Distal arthrogryposes: Subset of nonprogressive contractures without associated primary neurological or muscle disease affecting limb function
- Classic imaging appearance
  - Severe cases show no extremity movement
  - Occasional "roll" of fetal trunk
- Spectrum of involvement from several to all joints
- **Arthrogryposis is a description not a diagnosis**
- Over 150 conditions described with arthrogryposis as a feature
- Altered fetal movement common link in pathogenesis
  - Muscle abnormality
    - Myotonic dystrophy
    - Myasthenia gravis: Neonatal myasthenia in 12%
    - Amyoplasia
  - Neurological disease
    - Anterior horn cell damage
    - CNS malformations
  - Connective tissue defects
  - Mechanical limitation of movement
    - Oligohydramnios
    - Multiple gestation

Imaging Findings
<u>General Features</u>
- Best imaging clue: Lack of extremity motion

Arthrogryposis

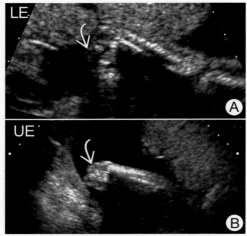

Arthrogryposis. Ultrasound images of upper (UE) and lower (LE) extremities show abnormal positioning. The limbs are held in extension with abnormal fixed flexion of the hand and foot (arrows). The extremity positions did not change during prolonged scanning.

Ultrasound Findings
- Odd extremity positioning
  - Extended legs
  - Flexed wrists
  - "Knotted" fingers
- Webbed joint spaces
- Polyhydramnios: Decreased fetal swallowing
- Pulmonary hypoplasia: Short ribs, lack of fetal breathing
- Short umbilical cord: Thought to relate to lack of fetal movement
- Some causes associated with intrauterine growth restriction (IUGR)

MR Findings
- May be performed for evaluation of brain
  - Agenesis of corpus callosum
  - Lissencephaly
  - Dandy-Walker

Imaging Recommendations
- Careful survey for associated anomalies
- Multiple structural anomalies and IUGR
  - Increased risk trisomy 18
- Upper extremity in "waiter's tip" position
  - Amyoplasia
- "Whistling" face with pursed lips on profile
  - Freeman-Sheldon syndrome
- Risk of respiratory difficulties at birth increased with
  - Polyhydramnios
  - Micrognathia
  - Thin ribs
  - Decreased fetal movements

Arthrogryposis

Differential Diagnosis: Specific features of some causative conditions

Trisomy 18
- Multiple structural anomalies
- "Classic" finger position (clenched hand with overlapping index finger)

Multiple Pterygium Syndrome
- Webbing across joints
- Cystic hygroma

Freeman-Sheldon Syndrome
- "Whistling" face: Mouth may be only few mm in diameter
- Scoliosis

Amyoplasia
- Upper extremity "waiter's tip" position

Pathology

General
- Genetics
  - 2% chromosomal abnormality
    - Trisomy 18, mosaic Trisomy 8
  - Autosomal dominant: Distal arthrogryposis
    - Some distal arthrogryposes map to chromosomes 9, 11
  - Autosomal recessive
    - Pena Shokeir **syndrome** (hereditary malformation motor neuron cells with specific neuropathological findings)
    - Scandinavian lethal congenital contractures
- Etiology-Pathogenesis
  - Destruction of anterior horn cells may be an underlying cause
  - Maximum sensitivity to hypoxia at 8 to 14 weeks gestation
- Epidemiology
  - 1:3,000 live births

Clinical Issues

Presentation
- Pena Shokeir diagnosed by 14 weeks
- Lethal Scandinavian type presents with hydrops and lower extremity malposition by 13 to 16 weeks

Treatment
- Genetic counseling: Offer karyotype
- Deliver at tertiary center: Risk of respiratory failure
- Vaginal delivery may be compromised by fixed extremity position

Prognosis
- Depends on
  - Number and severity of contractures
  - Associated anomalies/chromosomal disorders
- Ventilator dependence at birth $\Rightarrow$ poor prognosis
  - Rule out myasthenia gravis prior to withdrawal ventilatory support
    - Edrophonium chloride challenge test

Selected References
1. Sung SS et al: Mutations in genes encoding fast-twitch contractile proteins cause distal arthrogryposis syndromes. Am J Hum Genet 72:681-90, 2002
2. Krakowiak PA et al: A variant of Freeman-Sheldon syndrome maps to 11p15.5-pter. Am J Hum Genet 60:426-32, 1997
3. Bianchi DW et al: An approach to ventilator-dependent neonates with arthrogryposis. Pediatrics 94:682-6, 1994

Clubfoot/Rockerbottom Foot

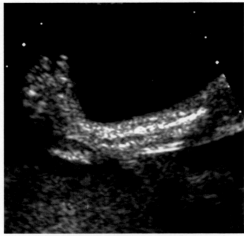

Clubfoot. Isolated clubfoot in a second trimester fetus. Longitudinal view of the lower extremity shows both the leg and inverted foot in the same view. Fetus had no other anomalies and karyotype was normal.

Key Facts
- Synonyms
  - Clubfoot: Talipes, talipes equinovarus, talipes valgus
  - Rockerbottom foot: Convex pes valgus, convex foot, vertical talus
- Definition
  - Clubfoot: **Abnormal relationship of foot/ankle to tibia/fibula**
  - Rockerbottom foot: Convex foot, dorsolateral dislocation of midfoot
  - Talipes = club foot
  - Valgus = bent outward, varus = bent inward
  - Equinus = plantar flexed
- Classic imaging appearance:
  - Clubfoot: Foot is abnormally oriented with regards to tibia and fubula
  - Rockerbottom foot: Foot shape is convex +/- clubfoot
- Difficult to tell exactly what kind of talipes on prenatal ultrasound
  - **Talipes equinovarus most common**
- **Highly associated with other anomalies**
- Associated with chromosome abnormalities
- **False positive and false negative diagnoses** common
- Often bilateral

Imaging Findings
General Features
- Best imaging clue
  - Clubfoot: Foot consistently seen deviated 90 degrees inward at ankle
  - Rockerbottom: Foot foreshortened and convex, like **"Persian slipper"**
Ultrasound Findings
- Clubfoot
  - **Long axis of foot in same plane as long axis of tibia and fibula**
    - Normal: Coronal view of lower leg ends in short axis of foot

Clubfoot/Rockerbottom Foot

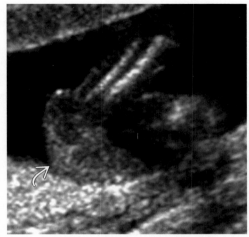

Rockerbottom foot. Rockerbottom foot in fetus with trisomy 18. Notice the convex position of the foot (arrow). This was a persistent finding and multiple other complex anomalies were also noted.

- o Talipes equinovarus: Foot plantar flexed (like horse hoof)
  - ▪ Medial deviation of foot and ankle
  - ▪ Foot length shortened since flexed
- o **60% with bilateral clubfeet**
- o **50% associated with other anomalies**, 50% isolated
  - ▪ 20% of associated anomalies not seen at time of first ultrasound
- Rockerbottom foot
  - o May be associated with clubfoot
  - o Foot hyperextended and convex on sagittal views
    - ▪ Foot length shortened since convex
  - o 70% bilateral
  - o **Rarely isolated**
- Clubfoot/rockerbottom foot common associations
  - o Fetal akinesia deformation sequence
    - ▪ Decreased fetal movement from any cause
    - ▪ Intrauterine growth restriction (IUGR), limb anomalies, pulmonary hypoplasia, depressed nose, polyhydramnios
  - o Chronic **oligohydramnios**
    - ▪ From any cause: Renal most common
  - o Abnormal nerve function or innervation
    - ▪ **Spina bifida**, spinal dysraphism
  - o Intrinsic abnormality of fetal musculature or connective tissue
    - ▪ Myotonic dystrophy
  - o **Trisomy 18**
    - ▪ Clubfoot in 23%
    - ▪ Rockerbottom foot in 10%
    - ▪ Other severe anomalies usually also seen

Imaging Recommendations
- Rule out transient foot position
  - o When isolated finding, consider follow-up

Clubfoot/Rockerbottom Foot

- **Three dimensional ultrasound** may be helpful
  - o **Allows for meticulous exam using multiplanar imaging**

Differential Diagnosis
Normal Foot Position
- **Fetus transiently holds foot inverted**
- Suspect if finding is mild and isolated
- Most common cause of **clubfoot false positive diagnosis (12%)**

Pathology
General
- Etiology-Pathogenesis
  - o **Normal development requires embryo movement**
    - Movement starts at 7-8 weeks
  - o Lack of movement from any cause
    - Extremity deformity/contractures
- Epidemiology
  - o Clubfoot
    - **1/1,000** diagnosed in utero
    - 60% bilateral, 40% unilateral
    - 50% associated with other abnormalities
  - o Rockerbottom foot
    - More rare, 1/100 clubfoot
    - 70% bilateral and likely associated with trisomy 18

Clinical Issues
Presentation
- Incidentally noted on routine ultrasound
- In association with other anomalies
Treatment
- Role of amniocentesis
  - o Controversial for isolated club foot 0-6% false negatives reported (other anomalies found after delivery)
    - Trisomy 18, trisomy 21, 47XXY, 47XXX missed cases reported
  - o Indicated when associated abnormalities seen
- Clubfoot
  - o **60% surgery**, 40% serial casts or no therapy necessary
- Rockerbottom foot
  - o Almost always need surgery
Prognosis
- Depends on karyotype and associated anomalies
- Isolated do well

Selected References
1. Bakalis S et al: Outcome of antenatally diagnosed talipes equinovarus in an unselected obstetric population. Ultrasound Obstet Gynecol 20:226-9, 2002
2. Malone FD et al: Isolated clubfoot diagnosed prenatally: Is karyotyping indicated? Obstet Gynecol 95:437-40, 2000
3. Shipp TD et al: The significance of prenatally identified isolated clubfoot: Is amniocentesis indicated? Am J Obstet Gynecol 178:600-2, 1998

Amniotic Band Syndrome

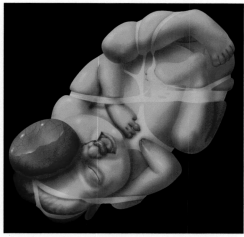

Amniotic band syndrome. Illustration shows various manifestations of amniotic band syndrome including constrictions, amputations, facial clefts, and a cephalocele.

Key Facts
- Synonyms: ADAM (**amniotic deformity, adhesion, mutilation**), amniotic band sequence, amniotic disruption complex
- Definition: Entrapment of fetal parts by disrupted amnion resulting in clefts, constrictions, and amputations
- Classic imaging appearance: Fetus with random, often bizarre appearing, **slash defects** affecting multiple body areas
- Early disruption more likely to produce major, often lethal malformations
  - Craniofacial
  - Body wall
- Later disruption often results in musculoskeletal deformities

Imaging Findings
General Features
- Best imaging clue: **Asymmetric distribution** of defects is hallmark of syndrome
- Defects may be isolated or multiple but not in specific pattern
Ultrasound Findings
- Bands in amniotic fluid appear as multiple thin membranes
  - May be difficult to discern especially in setting of oligohydramnios
- Face and head
  - **Facial clefts**
    - Do not conform to pattern of developmental clefts
    - Often oblique
    - Deformity of facial features often severe
  - Cephaloceles
    - Occur in area other than along sutures
  - Anencephaly
    - Asymmetric defect with portion of skull or brain remaining
  - Acrania

Amniotic Band Syndrome

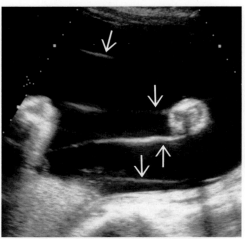

Amniotic band syndrome. Multiple thin membranes are identified within the amniotic fluid, some of which are wrapped around a fetal extremity (arrows).

- **Extremeties**
  - **Limb amputations**
    - Often fingers and toes
    - Easily missed if isolated
  - **Constriction with edema** of distal extremity
    - May lead to eventual amputation
  - Ring constrictions
  - Clubbed feet and hands
  - Pseudosyndactyly
    - Fusion of distal digits
- Thoracic and abdominal wall defects
- Oligohydramnios in some cases
  - Fluid leaks between amnion and chorion and is reabsorbed

Imaging Recommendations
- If unusual distribution of defects, look carefully for bands
  - May be tightly adherent and difficult to see
- **Color Doppler to assess flow** to affected extremity

Differential Diagnosis

Body Stalk Anomalies
- **Fetus adherent to placenta**
- **Absent umbilical cord**
- Scoliosis major finding

Developmental Body Defects
- All have **defined anatomic distributions** from embryologic development
- Cephalocele
  - Occipital and frontal
- Cleft lip
  - Unilateral, bilateral, or midline (not oblique)
- Gastroschisis
  - Right of midline adjacent to cord insertion

Amniotic Band Syndrome

- Omphalocele
  - Herniation into base of umbilical cord

Amniotic Sheets
- Amnion wrapping around synechiae
- Thick at base with free edge
- Fetus freely mobile

Chorioamniotic Separation
- No entrapment of fetal parts

Pathology
General
- General Path Comments
  - Ruptured amnion does not always lead to amniotic band syndrome
  - Not associated with aneuploidy
- Etiology-Pathogenesis: (Incompletely understood)
  - Proposed (does not completely explain some cases)
    - Disruption of amnion
    - **Chorionic side of amnion is "sticky"**
    - Entrapment of fetal part
    - Vascular constriction $\Rightarrow$ edema $\Rightarrow$ deformity or amputation
  - Described risk factors: Amniocentesis, drugs (methadone, LSD), Ehlers-Danlos syndrome, epidermolysis bullosa
- Epidemiology
  - 1:1,200-1,500 live births

Clinical Issues
Presentation
- Evaluation of major malformation
  - May be detected in 1st trimester
- Incidental finding for minor extremity deformity

Treatment
- Termination offered for major defects
- Successful in utero lysis of bands for at-risk extremity reported

Prognosis
- Defects range from minor to lethal
- No recurrence risk

Selected References
1. Tadmor OP et al: Limb amputation in amniotic band syndrome: Serial ultrasonographic and Doppler observations. Ultrasound Obstet Gynecol 10:312-5, 1997
2. Quintero RA et al: In utero lysis of amniotic bands. Ultrasound Obstet Gynecol 10:316-20, 1997
3. Mahony BS et al: The amniotic band syndrome: antenatal sonographic diagnosis and potential pitfalls. Am J Obstet Gynecol 152:63-8, 1985

Radial Ray Malformation

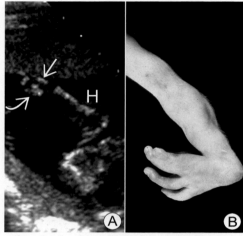

Radial ray malformation in a fetus with Trisomy 18. (A) Image of the left upper extremity shows a normal humerus (H). There is a single, short, forearm bone (arrow) with the hand held in fixed flexion (curved arrow). (B) Photograph confirms US findings. Also note absent thumb and syndactyly of 2nd and 3rd digits.

Key Facts

- Synonyms: Radial ray hypoplasia, radial ray aplasia
- Definition: Spectrum of anomalies including absence or hypoplasia of
  - Radius
  - Radial carpal bones
  - Thumb
  - +/- malposition or "fingerization" of thumb
- Classic imaging appearance: **Single forearm bone, abnormal hand positioning**
- Categories of disease manifesting radial aplasia
  - **Chromosome/single gene disorders**
    - Trisomy 18
    - Holt-Oram: Bilateral, asymmetric, upper extremity defects associated with congenital heart disease
    - Fanconi anemia
    - Thrombocytopenia absent radius (TAR)
  - **Teratogen exposure**
    - Valproic acid
    - Thalidomide
  - **Syndromes**
    - VACTERL
    - Cornelia de Lange (facial anomalies, limb reduction, microcephaly)
    - Nager: Acrofacial dysostosis
    - Omphalocele-radial-ray (ORR) complex

Imaging Findings

<u>General Features</u>
- Best imaging clue: Single forearm bone
<u>Ultrasound Findings</u>
- Vary with type and cause

Radial Ray Malformation

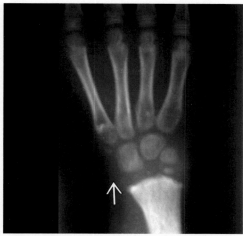

Radial ray malformation. Radiograph of the wrist of a child with radial ray anomaly. There is single forearm bone with absent thumb and radial metacarpals. Note absence of the scaphoid, trapezium and trapezoid (STT) (arrow - where normal STT should be located).

- Hand is fully formed by 14 weeks
- Nomograms exist for length all long bones
- Multiple anomalies increase likelihood of VACTERL or chromosome defect

<u>Imaging Recommendations</u>
- Fetal echocardiogram
  - o Cardiac defect in 95% Holt Oram: Atrial septal defect (ASD), ventricular septal defect (VSD)
  - o VACTERL association: C = cardiac lesion
- Careful search for other structural anomaly
  - o 86% **patients** with hypoplastic thumbs have other anomaly
  - o Fetal incidence not known
- Monitor growth
  - o **Intra-uterine growth restriction (IUGR) ⇒ chromosome abnormality more likely**

Differential Diagnosis
<u>Short Limbed Skeletal Dysplasia</u>
- All long bones affected (to variable degree)
- Usually shortening rather than absence
- Often associated skull or spine abnormalities
- Often abnormal mineralization

<u>Amputation Defects</u>
- Look for amniotic bands
- Affects multiple areas

Pathology
<u>General</u>
- Genetics
  - o Autosomal dominant

Radial Ray Malformation

- - Holt Oram (increases in severity in succeeding generations)
  - Nager syndrome
  o Autosomal recessive
    - Fanconi anemia
    - TAR
  o X-linked recessive forms exist but are extremely rare
- Etiology-Pathogenesis
  o Embryology
  o Damage to apical ectoderm of limb bud between 6 and 12 weeks
    - Vascular anomaly
    - Local toxins: Maternal diabetes, valproic acid
    - Maternal infection
- Epidemiology
  o 1:30,000 live births
  o Bilateral in 50%

Clinical Issues
Presentation
- Should be detected on routine anatomic survey at 16 to 18 weeks
Natural History
- Depends on associated anomalies
Treatment
- Genetic counseling
- Offer karyotype
  o Aneuploidy
  o Fanconi anemia
    - Chromosomes must be studied after exposure to diepoxybutane
- Exclude maternal diabetes
- Examine parents for subtle defects
  o **Holt-Oram shows anticipation** (i.e., increasing severity of defects in successive generations)
- Consider cordocentesis if family history of TAR
  o Thrombocytopenia, aplastic anemia
- Risk of dystocia with flexion deformities at elbow
- Rare lesions: Require referral to specialist centers for reconstructive surgery
  o Classification system developed to allow
    - Tracking of occurrence
    - Follow-up of treatment
Prognosis
- Depends on underlying cause
  o Trisomy 18: Dismal
  o Triphalangeal thumb: If isolated, can be surgically corrected at 1-2 years
- Recurrence risk relates to underlying condition

Selected References
1. De Smet L et al: Classification for congenital anomalies of the hand: The IFSSH classification and the JSSH modification. Genet Couns 13:331-8, 2002
2. De Kerviler E et al: The clinical and radiological features of Fanconi's anemia. Clin Radiol 55:340-5, 2000
3. James MA et al: Characteristics of patients with hypoplastic thumbs. J Hand Surg 21:104-13, 1996

Polydactyly

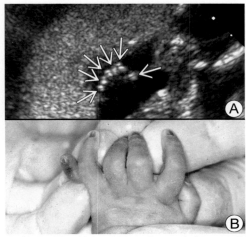

Polydactyly. (A) Ultrasound and (B) postpartum photograph show postaxial polydactyly of the hand. Note the fingers are curved so more than one phalanx is seen in each digit (arrows). This can make counting very difficult. Multiple views should be obtained to confirm.

Key Facts
- Definition: One or more extra digits occurring in one of two patterns
  - **Preaxial**: Radial or tibial side
  - **Postaxial**: Ulnar or fibular side
- Classic imaging appearance: Six or more digits on one or both hands or feet
- Postaxial most common
  - 10 x more common in Blacks
- Described in over 100 syndromes

Imaging Findings
General Features
- Best imaging clue: Need to confirm in both axial and coronal views
  - **Oblique views may give erroneous appearance** of polydactyly
Ultrasound Findings
- Extra digit may be small or angulated
- May be fleshy nubbin without bone
  - Difficult to see in utero
  - Often missed
- Postaxial
  - Extra digit in same plane as normal digits
  - May attach directly to normal digit (bifid digit)
- Preaxial
  - Extra digit proximally located
- **Role for 3D ultrasound**
  - Better able to delineate anatomy
  - Aids in diagnosis
Imaging Recommendations
- **Count and recount**
  - Easy to both under and over diagnose

Polydactyly

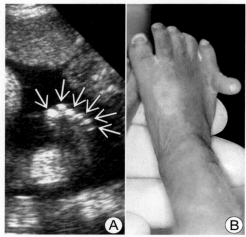

Polydactyly in a fetus with trisomy 13. (A) Ultrasound and (B) postpartum photograph show postaxial polydactyly of the foot (arrows).

- o **Make sure hands (or feet) are not together**
    - ▪ Erroneous appearance of polydactyly
- o **Confirm in both axial and coronal planes**
- Careful scanning for other abnormalities and syndromes
- Cardiac echo if other abnormalities identified

Differential Diagnosis: Conditions with Polydactyly
Trisomy 13
- Holoprosencephaly
- Cystic renal disease
- Cardiac defects

Meckel-Gruber Syndrome
- Encephalocele
- Renal cystic dysplasia
- Polydactyly

Short Rib Polydactyly
- Small chest
- Short extremities
- Polydactyly

Ellis-van Creveld (Chondroectodermal Dysplasia)
- Disorder of endochondral ossification
- Small chest
- Polydactyly
- Cardiac defects
- High incidence in Amish population

Smith-Lemli-Opitz Syndrome
- Inborn error in cholesterol metabolism
- Cardiac defects
- Microcephaly
- Cleft palate
- Cryptorchidism

Polydactyly

Carpenter Syndrome
- Craniosynostosis resulting in oxycephaly
- Preaxial polydactyly
- Syndactyly
- Cardiac defects

Pathology
General
- General Path Comments
  - Triphalangeal ("finger-like") thumb considered part of preaxial spectrum
  - Syndactyly may be associated in some cases
- Genetics
  - Variable according to syndrome
  - Isolated: Majority are familial with variable inheritance patterns
    - Most autosomal dominant
- Epidemiology
  - Postaxial
    - 1:3,000 Caucasian
    - 1:300 Blacks
  - Preaxial (less common)
    - 1:10,000
    - No racial difference

Gross Pathologic, Surgical Features
- Variable amounts of development
  - Soft tissue only (skin tag)
  - Variable amounts of phalangeal development and function

Clinical Issues
Presentation
- Minor finding with other major malformations
- Incidental finding if isolated

Treatment
- **All fetuses should be karyotyped**
- Thorough family history
- Genetic counseling regarding syndromes
- Resection of extra digit varies in complexity
  - Without bone, may be done in nursery
  - With bone, often wait until 1-2 years old
    - May require joint reconstruction or tendon transfer

Prognosis
- Variable according to syndrome
- Isolated excellent

Selected References
1. Kos M et al: Limb deformities and three-dimensional ultrasound. J Perinat Med 30:40-7, 2002
2. Bromley B et al: Isolated polydactyly: Prenatal diagnosis and perinatal outcome. Prenat Diagn 20:905-8, 2000
3. Zimmer EZ et al: Fetal polydactyly diagnosis during early pregnancy: Clinical applications. Am J Obstet Gynecol 183:755-8, 2000

Caudal Regression Sequence

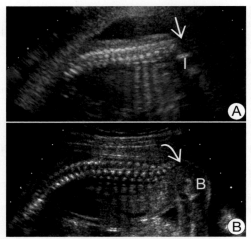

Caudal regression sequence. Sagittal spine in affected fetus (A) compared to normal (B). Note abrupt termination of spine (arrow) superior to iliac blade (I). In the normal fetus spine tapers to a point (curved arrow) at the level of the fetal buttocks (B).

Key Facts
- Synonyms: Caudal aplasia, caudal dysplasia
- Definition: Variable degree agenesis/disruption distal neural tube
- Classic imaging appearance: Absent sacrum +/- absent distal lumbar vertebrae
- Associated with
  - Gastrointestinal (GI)/genitourinary (GU) anomalies
  - Lower extremity dysfunction
- **Maternal diabetes** significant risk factor

Imaging Findings
General Features
- Best imaging clue: **Absent sacrum with hypoplastic lower extremities** is diagnostic
Ultrasound Findings
- Abrupt termination of the spine
- Short trunk
- Clubfeet
- Lower extremity contractures: **"Buddha" pose**
- Normal to increased amniotic fluid
- Associated with wide range of anomalies
  - GI: Anorectal/duodenal atresia
  - GU: Cystic renal dysplasia, dilated bladder, hydronephrosis
  - CNS: Spina bifida
  - Cardiovascular system (CVS)
MR Findings
- Theoretical benefit for associated anomalies especially with maternal obesity

Caudal Regression Sequence

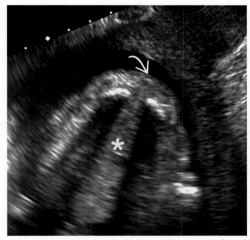

Caudal regression sequence. Transvaginal axial scan at the level of iliac blades shows absence of the sacrum (curved arrow). Note increased through transmission of sound (*).

Imaging Recommendations
- Normal sagittal spine tapers to a point at the fetal buttock
- Beware "tapering" distal spine, **can taper when it terminates not just at sacrum!**
- Coronal section shows ribs, count down lumbar segments to show five present
- **Axial view at level iliac crests best** to show sacrum
- Sacrum not well ossified until mid second trimester: **Mild cases easily missed**
- Fetal echocardiography: Strong association with cardiovascular anomalies
  - Should be routine with maternal insulin-dependent diabetes

Differential Diagnosis
Myelomeningocele
- Ossification centers present
- Posterior elements splayed
- Look for sac
- Associated with Arnold-Chiari defect
  - Obliteration of cisterna magna
  - "Banana" cerebellum
  - "Lemon" sign: Invariably resolves by 34 weeks
VACTERL: Combination of Anomalies
- Vertebral
- Anorectal
- Cardiac
- Tracheoesophageal fistula
- Renal
- Limb
- **Not associated with maternal diabetes**

Caudal Regression Sequence

Pathology
General
- Genetics
  - Occasional familial cases
- Etiology-Pathogenesis
  - Distal neural tube fails to form
- Epidemiology
  - M:F = 1:1
  - 1:5/100,000
  - 1% of infants born to diabetic mothers have caudal regression sequence (CRS)
  - 12-16% infants with CRS have diabetic mothers
    - Poor glycemic control thought to be etiologic factor

Gross Pathologic, Surgical Features
- Spectrum
  - Abnormal sacrum with normal lower extremities
  - Absent sacrum
  - Abnormal lower lumbar spine, occasional T spine involvement
  - Clubfeet
  - Flexion deformities hips/knees
  - "Cross legged tailor" or "buddha" pose
  - Decreased or absent lower extremity movement
- Sirenomelia no longer considered part of this sequence
  - Fused lower extremities
  - Renal agenesis
  - Anhydramnios
  - Vascular defect as cause
  - Lethal

Clinical Issues
Presentation
- Described as early as 11 weeks gestation

Treatment
- Maternal diabetes testing
- Fetal echocardiography
- Orthopedic surgery for clubfeet/contractures

Prognosis
- Similar to high/mid lumbar myelomeningocele
- Neurogenic bladder
- Motor deficit > sensory
- High mortality due to associated anomalies

Selected References
1. Subtil D et al: Early detection of caudal regression syndrome: Specific interest and findings in three cases. Eur J Obstet Gynecol Reprod Biol 80:109-12, 1998
2. Adra A et al: Caudal regression syndrome: Etiopathogenesis, prenatal diagnosis and perinatal management. Obstet Gynecol Surv 49:508-16, 1994
3. Twickler D et al: Caudal regression versus sirenomelia. J Ultrasound Med 12:323-30, 1993

PocketRadiologist®
Obstetrics
Top 100 Diagnoses

CORD

Single Umbilical Artery

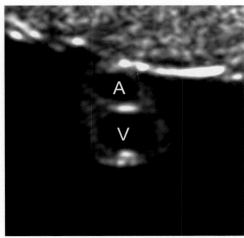

Single umbilical artery. A transverse view of a free loop of umbilical cord in amniotic fluid shows only two vessels, a single umbilical artery (A) and an umbilical vein (V). Note the diameter of the umbilical artery is greater than 50% that of the umbilical vein.

Key Facts
- Synonyms: Absent umbilical artery, two vessel cord
- Definition: **Congenital absence of right or left umbilical artery** resulting in single umbilical artery (SUA) + umbilical vein (UV) in umbilical cord
- Classic imaging appearance: **Only two vessels**, instead of three, seen in all views of umbilical cord
- Documentation of number of vessels in cord is part of routine exam
- Usually, **common isolated incidental finding**
- Associated with **chromosome abnormalities** when not isolated
  - Trisomy 18
  - Trisomy 13
  - **Not trisomy 21**
- Increased incidence of intrauterine growth restriction (**IUGR**)

Imaging Findings
General Features
- Best imaging clue: Two-vessel umbilical cord seen in amniotic fluid and within fetal pelvis
Ultrasound Findings
- Transverse and longitudinal views of umbilical cord clearly shows only 2 vessels (SUA + UV)
- **Intra-abdominal segment is also absent**
  - Umbilical arteries travel around fetal bladder and insert into iliac arteries
  - **Transverse view of fetal bladder is best view**
  - Easily seen with **color or power Doppler**
  - Best way to tell if right or left UA is absent once SUA is suspect
- **Less coiled** than normal cord
  - On longitudinal views, SUA lies parallel to UV

Single Umbilical Artery

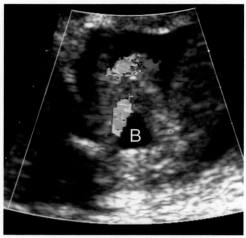

Single umbilical artery. Transverse image of fetal pelvis with color Doppler shows only one umbilical artery (color flow) adjacent to fetal bladder (B).

- **SUA is larger** than UA in a normal cord
  - > 50% diameter of vein
    - Normal is < 50%
    - All blood volume vs half volume in UA of 3 vessel cord
- **70% are absent left UA**
  - No difference in outcome or associated anomalies
- Associations with SUA
  - Trisomy 18 (T18)
  - Trisomy 13 (T13)
  - **IUGR (15%)**
  - **Renal anomalies**
    - Unilateral renal agenesis
    - Sirenomelia: Always has SUA
  - Velamentous cord insertion
  - Twin reversed arterial perfusion sequence

Imaging Recommendations
- Color Doppler for all cases
- If suspect SUA in cord, look for UA on transverse pelvis views to confirm
- Look carefully for fetal anomalies
  - Renal anomalies
  - Markers for T18, T13
- **Follow-up ultrasound for growth**

Differential Diagnosis

Hypoplastic Umbilical Artery
- Small right or left umbilical artery
  - Intra-amniotic and intra-abdominal UA is hypoplastic
- > 50% difference in size between right and left UA
- Within spectrum of SUA with same associations
- Doppler shows discordant blood flow
  - Increased resistance in smaller artery

Single Umbilical Artery

- ▪ Higher systolic/diastolic ratio

<u>Fused UA Near Placental Insertion</u>
- Right and left UA may normally fuse within 3 cm of placenta
- Longer segments of fusion may mimic SUA
- Probably not associated with other abnormalities

Pathology
<u>General</u>
- Etiology-Pathogenesis
  - o Embryology: Proposed etiologies
    - ▪ Atrophy of a previously normal UA
    - ▪ Persistence of vitelline artery (most likely with sirenomelia)
- Epidemiology
  - o Prevalence: **0.63% newborn infants**
  - o Higher prevalence in Caucasians

Clinical Issues
<u>Presentation</u>
- Usually incidental isolated finding
  - o No need for amniocentesis
  - o Follow up for growth
- Secondary finding associated with other anomalies
  - o Consider amniocentesis
<u>Treatment</u>
- Postnatal ultrasound of kidneys if not seen well on prenatal scan
<u>Prognosis</u>
- Excellent when isolated
- Poor when associated with severe anomalies, T18, T13

Selected References
1. Chow JS et al: Frequency and nature of structural anomalies in fetuses with single umbilical arteries. J Ultrasound Med 17:765-8, 1998
2. Catanzarite VA et al: Prenatal diagnosis of the two-vessel cord: implications for patient counseling and obstetric management. Ultrasound Obstet Gynecol 5:98-105, 1995
3. Parrilla BV et al: The clinical significance of single umbilical artery as an isolated finding on prenatal ultrasound. Obstet Gynecol 85:570-2, 1995

Umbilical Cord Cyst

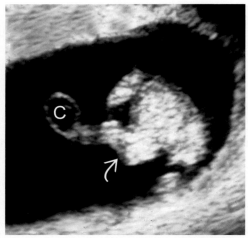

Umbilical cord cyst. First trimester ultrasound of the umbilical cord shows a small cyst (C). Note that the cyst occurs at the same time as physiologic bowel herniation (curved arrow). This cyst resolved, and fetal outcome was normal.

Key Facts
- Definition: Pseudocysts or epithelial-lined true cysts of umbilical cord
- Classic imaging appearance: **Round cyst or cysts** associated with umbilical cord (UC)
- **Pseudocysts more common**
  - Associated with edema or degeneration of Wharton's jelly (gelatinous stroma which covers cord)
- **True cysts may be associated with fetal structural anomalies**
  - Allantoic
  - Omphalomesenteric duct
  - Urachal
- Pseudocysts and true cysts are often sonographically identical
- **Usually an incidental finding** that resolves
- Seen most commonly in 1st or 2nd trimester
  - In 1st trimester often seen at time of UC coiling

Imaging Findings
General Features
- Best imaging clue: One or more cysts associated with UC
Ultrasound Findings
- Cyst or cysts, with or without internal echoes
- Multiple cysts tend to cluster
- More commonly **located at fetal or placental end of UC**
  - Mid-cord unusual
- **Allantoic cysts**
  - Located near fetus
  - Caused by communication between bladder and UC via **patent urachus**
    - Communication may be visible with careful imaging
  - **May grow** and cause compression of cord

Umbilical Cord Cyst

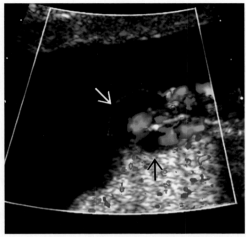

Umbilical cord cyst. Two cysts are seen at the placental origin of the umbilical cord (arrows). They are eccentric to cord vessels and probably represent pseudocysts. No fetal anomalies were seen, and pregnancy outcome was normal.

- o Color Doppler shows UC vessels surround cyst
  - ▪ **Cyst is in center of vessels**
- **Pseudocyst**
  - o Variable but stable size
  - o May be multiple and clustered
  - o **Cyst is eccentric to vessels**
- **Omphalomesenteric duct cyst**
  - o Resembles pseudocyst
  - o May be **associated with other anomalies**
    - ▪ Intraabdominal mesenteric cyst
    - ▪ Umbilical cord polyps
    - ▪ Omphalocele
    - ▪ Diaphragmatic hernia
    - ▪ Cardiac defects
    - ▪ Spina bifida
    - ▪ Trisomy 21 (T21)
- **First trimester cysts**
  - o Often resolve by 2nd trimester
  - o Probably pseudocysts
  - o **Associated with coiling of UC and physiologic bowel herniation**

Imaging Recommendations
- Look for associated anomalies, markers for T21
- Note location of cyst compared to cord vessels
  - o Central vs. eccentric
- Follow up to see if cyst is growing

Differential Diagnosis

Normal First Trimester Yolk Sac
- Unlike cord cyst, yolk sac is located outside of amniotic sac

Umbilical Cord Cyst

Umbilical Vein Varix
- Focally distended umbilical vein
- Flow on color Doppler

Resolving UC Hematoma
- History of cordocentesis or significant trauma
- Changes appearance over time
  o Echogenic → cystic

Pathology
General
- Etiology-Pathogenesis
  o Pseudocysts: Suggested etiology
    ▪ Increased hydrostatic pressure in UC from coiling and midgut herniation
    ▪ Leads to fluid transfer into **Wharton's jelly** with cyst formation from mucoid or cystic degeneration
  o True cysts: Suggested etiology
    ▪ Embryonic remnants of allantois, omphalomesenteric, and vitelline ducts

Microscopic Features
- True cysts are lined by epithelium

Clinical Issues
Presentation
- Incidentally noted during 1st or 2nd trimester exam
- In association with other anomalies

Natural History
- Most first trimester cysts resolve
- Pseudocysts resolve or remain stable
- Allantoic cysts may grow if associated with patent urachus

Treatment
- Usually none necessary
- If cyst is compromising cord, then early delivery is considered
- Consider amniocentesis when associated with anomalies and T21 markers

Prognosis
- Excellent when isolated

Selected References
1.   Sepulveda W et al: Clinical significance of first trimester umbilical cord cysts. J Ultrasound Med 18:95-9, 1999
2.   Sepulveda W et al: Prenatal diagnosis of umbilical cord pseudocyst. Ultrasound Obstet Gynecol 4:147-50, 1994
3.   Persutte WH et al: Antenatal diagnosis of fetal patent urachus. J Ultrasound Med 7:399-403, 1988

Cord Doppler: Normal/Abnormal

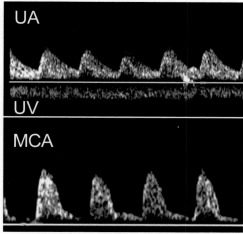

Cord Doppler normal. Examples of normal third trimester appearance of UA, UV and MCA waveforms. UA has continuous antegrade flow in diastole, UV has "flat," non-pulsatile flow. MCA is high resistance with little antegrade diastolic flow.

Key Facts
- Definition: Measurement of velocity and direction of flow in umbilical artery (UA) and vein (UV)
- Classic imaging appearance
  - Normal UA
    - Low resistance waveform: Continuous antegrade diastolic flow
    - No notch
  - Normal UV
    - Continuous flow: "Flat" waveform
- Doppler effect: Sound frequency changes as it reflects off moving objects
  - In this context the moving object is blood in umbilical vessels
- Interpretation requires understanding of **normal placental flow**
  - Deoxygenated blood leaves fetus via UAs
  - UAs branch on placental surface, enter chorionic villi (CV)
  - CV bathed in "pool" of maternal blood: Intervillus space
    - Trophoblastic invasion of spiral artery walls
  - Oxygen exchange occurs at this level
  - CV venules join to form umbilical vein (UV)
  - UV ⇒ ductus venosus (DV) ⇒ inferior vena cava (IVC)
  - DV component of IVC flow is oxygen rich
    - Shunted across foramen ovale (FO) ⇒ LA ⇒ LV ⇒ aorta
- When placental resistance (PR) increases ⇒ change in UA waveform
  - LV pressure changes in attempt to overcome PR
  - "Kick back" along circuit LA ⇒ RA ⇒ DV ⇒ IVC ⇒ UV
- **UV is last place to change** with abnormal umbilical circulation

Imaging Findings
General Features
- Flow "quantified" by ratios: Not angle dependent
  - **SD ratio**: Peak systolic velocity (PSV)/End diastolic velocity (EDV)

Cord Doppler: Normal/Abnormal

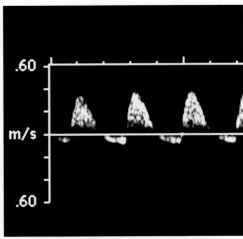

Cord Doppler abnormal. UA tracing showing REDF. Corresponding MCA Doppler showed low resistance indicating "head sparing" redistribution of flow. BPP was scored as 0/10. Infant was delivered by crash C-section immediately following this study.

- o **Resistive Index** (RI): PSV-EDV/PSV
  - ▪ RI = 1 with absent (AEDF) or reversed end diastolic flow (REDF)
- o **Pulsatility index** (PI): PSV-EDV/Time averaged velocity (TAV)
  - ▪ Accounts for flow throughout cardiac cycle
  - ▪ Includes reversed flow

Imaging Recommendations
- **Measure in consistent location**
  - o Cord insertion site: Highest resistance
  - o Placental insertion site: Lowest resistance
  - o Best to measure in free floating loop
- **In multifetal gestations, measure at cord insertion site**
  - o Ensures reliable serial measurements in individual fetuses
  - o Avoids variability due to site of measurement
- Look for signs placental insufficiency
  - o See " IUGR: Asymmetric"
- Confirm abnormal findings
  - o **Look at the waveform**: Tendency to measure "something" even when AEDF
- Do not do Doppler in normally grown fetuses
  - o All management data based on high risk pregnancy
  - o Cannot be applied to the general population

Differential Diagnosis
Pregnancy < 16 Weeks Gestation
- UA REDF **normal**
  - o Intervillous space not formed

Fetal Breathing
- Umbilical vein pulsation **not** linked to end diastole

Cord Doppler: Normal/Abnormal

Pathology
General
- Normal placentation
  - 1st trimester: Mesenchymal villi $\Rightarrow 1^0$, 2^0, 3^0 stem villi
  - 2nd trimester: Branching angiogenesis
    - 10-15 generations intermediate villi
  - 3rd trimester: Non-branching angiogenesis
    - Intermediate villi sprout **many** terminal villi
- Abnormal placentation $\Rightarrow$ failed/abnormal branching
  - Small muscular arteries obliterated in tertiary villi
- Epidemiology
  - Abnormal Doppler occurs with
    - IUGR: 10% of pregnancies
    - Aneuploidy

Clinical Issues
Presentation
- Placental insufficiency presents in second trimester
- **Uterine** artery Doppler may allow early selection of at-risk group
  - Intervention to prevent/decrease placental vascular disease

Treatment & Prognosis
- > 30 weeks: Abnormal Doppler contributes to decision to deliver
- **Dilemma** in second trimester
  - Risk of hostile intrauterine environment
  - Risks of extreme prematurity
- AEDF
  - 30% improve with bed rest, control maternal disease
  - Improvement occurs in 24-48 hours
  - Supports continuation of pregnancy in second trimester
- REDF
  - Quantified by ratio highest amplitude forward (A)/maximum reverse flow (B)
  - A/B ratio > 4.3, with absent venous pulsation in free loop may support expectant management of REDF in second trimester
- Normal Doppler reassuring for normal fetoplacental circulation
  - Anomalies/syndromes determine outcome even if Doppler normal
- Adverse perinatal outcome: 4 fold increase with intra-uterine growth retardation (IUGR)
  - IUGR + abnormal Doppler additional 4-8 fold increase
- **Perinatal Mortality**
  - AEDF: 8.9 %
  - REDF: 35.7 %
    - Associated with **fetal demise** within 1-7 days
- Arterial Doppler: "Tip of the iceberg"
  - Addition of venous Doppler $\Rightarrow$ more information on fetal response
  - More information $\Rightarrow$ better decision making

Selected References
1. Alfirevic Z et al: Doppler ultrasonography in high-risk pregnancies: Systematic review with meta-analysis. Am J Obstet Gynecol 172:1379-87, 1995
2. Forouzan I et al: Absence of end-diastolic flow in the umbilical artery: A review. Obstet Gynecol Surv 50:219-27, 1995
3. Tulzer G et al: Doppler in non-immune hydrops fetalis. Ultrasound Obstet Gynecol (Vol.):279-83, 1994

PocketRadiologist®
Obstetrics
Top 100 Diagnoses

PLACENTA/CERVIX

Placenta Previa

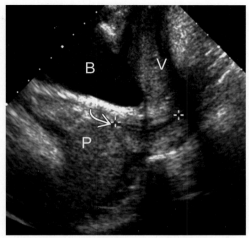

Placenta previa. Transperineal ultrasound of a complete placenta previa. The placenta (P) completely covers internal cervical os (arrow). Calipers measure cervical length. Note how the collapsed vagina (V) and partially filled bladder (B) serve as acoustic windows.

Key Facts
- Synonym: Low-lying placenta
- Definition: Abnormal placental implantation in lower uterine segment
- Classic imaging appearance: Placenta completely or partially covers internal cervical os
- Placenta previa may be **complete, marginal, or partial**
- **Low-lying placenta** often seen before 20 weeks and resolves by 34 weeks
- Patients most often present with **painless vaginal bleeding**
- Best diagnosed with careful transvaginal ultrasound (TVUS) or transperineal ultrasound (TPUS)
- Associated with life threatening placenta **accreta/percreta in 5%**

Imaging Findings
General Features
- Best imaging clue: Transabdominal view suggests placenta located in lower uterine segment, TVUS or TPUS confirms placenta previa
Ultrasound Findings
- **Accurate placental location** part of every 2nd and 3rd trimester exam
- Sonographer may notice "floating" presenting part in 3rd trimester
  - Increased soft tissue between fetal head and cervix
- **Complete previa**
  - Total coverage of cervical internal os
  - May be **central or asymmetric** in relation to cervix
  - **Almost never resolves** with advancing pregnancy
- **Partial and marginal previa**
  - Partial: Inferior edge of placenta partially covers internal os
  - Marginal: Placenta covers part of cervix but not internal os
  - May be **difficult to tell difference** between partial and marginal
  - **May resolve** with advancing pregnancy

Placenta Previa

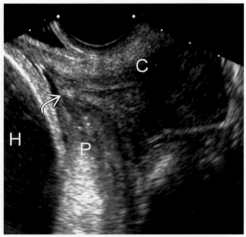

Placenta previa. Marginal/partial placenta previa in a third trimester patient with bleeding. Transvaginal ultrasound shows inferior edge of posterior placenta (P) located at internal cervical os (arrow). (C-cervix, H-fetal head).

- Low-lying placenta
  - Common before 20 weeks and **most resolve by 34 weeks**
  - Inferior edge within 2-3 cm of internal os
- Placenta previa and placenta acreta/percreta
  - Increased risk when multiple prior cesarean sections + anterior previa
  - Look for **intact myometrial zone** between placenta and bladder

MR Findings
- Mid sagittal planes are best
- Placenta location and relationship to cervix easily seen

Imaging Recommendations
- Transvaginal ultrasound technique for placenta previa
  - **Insert probe carefully with direct visualization**
  - Find midline sagittal plane and identify inferior edge of placenta
  - Measure **distance between placenta and internal os**
- **Transperineal/translabial technique** for placenta previa
  - Preferred method in **actively bleeding patients**
  - Elevate maternal hips to minimize artifact from bowel
  - Cover 3-5 MHz sector probe and place on perineum (labia minora)
  - Use collapsed vagina as acoustic window to cervix
  - Identify edge of placenta and measure distance to internal os

Differential Diagnosis

Overly Distended Bladder
- Mimics abnormally elongated cervix
  - Normally implanted placenta appears as previa
- Have **patient void** and repeat exam

Lower Uterine Segment Contraction
- Similar to overdistended bladder
- Usually resolves with time
- Note thick myometrium

- TVUS can often differentiate between cervix and contraction

Placenta Abruption

- Hematoma may be isoechoic with placenta and cover cervix
- Patient presents with bleeding (same as with previa)
- Power Doppler can help differentiate hematoma vs placenta
  - Slow flow in placenta and retro-placental vessels
  - No flow in hematoma

Pathology

General

- Etiology-Pathogenesis
  - Implantation of blastocyst in lower uterine segment (LUS)
    - Endometrial damage, poor endometrial blood supply
  - **Low-lying and marginal previas often resolve**
    - LUS grows later in pregnancy and "pulls" placenta up
  - Trophotropism
    - Placenta "dies" away in areas of poor blood supply (i.e., LUS)
    - Placenta "grows" in areas of better supply (i.e., upper uterus)
- Epidemiology
  - Incidence varies with gestational age at diagnosis and parity
    - 5% of cases between 15-16 weeks
    - 0.5% at term (only 1:1,500 nulliparous)
    - 90% low-lying placenta resolve
    - 5% with associated accreta, percreta, increta
  - **High risk patients**
    - Advanced maternal age, multiparity
    - Prior placenta previa, cesarean section, suction curettage
    - Smoking, cocaine use

Clinical Issues

Presentation

- Painless vaginal bleeding, usually in 3rd trimester
- Incidentally noted on ultrasound

Treatment

- Significant bleeding treated with bed rest/hospitalization
- Conservative management as long as possible to extend pregnancy
- Delivery by **cesarean section** for majority of cases
- Minority of marginal previas may be delivered vaginally
  - Fetal head may compress placenta during delivery
  - "Double set-up" so emergency cesarean if necessary

Prognosis

- **If previa is present at 34 weeks then it probably will not resolve**
- Excellent with appropriate management
- Maternal mortality < 1%

Selected References

1. Smith RS et al: Transvaginal ultrasonography for all placentas that appear to be low-lying or over the internal cervical os. Ultrasound Obstet Gynecol 9:22-4, 1997
2. Laurie MR et al: The use of second-trimester transvaginal sonography to predict placenta previa. Ultrasound Obstet Gynecol 8:337-40, 1996
3. Wing DA et al: Management of symptomatic placenta previa; a randomized, controlled trial of inpatient versus outpatient expectant management. Am J Obstet Gynecol 175:806-11, 1996

Placental Abruption

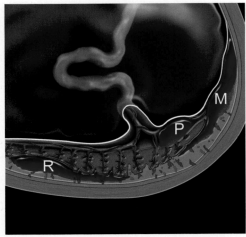

Placental abruption. Drawing of common sites of periplacental hemorrhage. Marginal abruption (M) occurs at the placenta edge. Retroplacental abruption (R) and preplacental hemorrhage (P) are less common.

Key Facts

- Synonym: Abruptio placenta
- Definition: Premature separation of placenta before birth
- Classic imaging appearance: Placental hematoma seen although appearance varies with size, location, and age of bleed
- Categorized by location as **retroplacental, marginal, pre-placental**
- Marginal abruption most common
- Retroplacental abruption most dangerous and difficult to diagnose
- Abruption is a **clinical diagnosis** and ultrasound may be negative
- Patients commonly present with bleeding and pain in third trimester
- Complicates **1% of all pregnancies**
- Most common cause of intrapartum fetal death

Imaging Findings

General Features
- Best imaging clue: **Placenta detached from myometrium** secondary to hypoechoic retroplacental or marginal hematoma

Ultrasound Findings
- Variable ultrasound findings depending on age, size, and location of bleed
  - Acute hematoma
    - Isoechoic to placenta or heterogeneous
    - **May mimic placenta**
  - Subacute hematoma
    - More complex and hypoechoic
  - Resolving hematoma
    - Liquefies: Sonolucent
- Marginal placental abruption
  - Blood in subchorionic space
  - **Most common type** of abruption
    - 91% of abruptions < 20 weeks

Placental Abruption

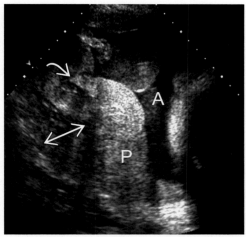

Placental Abruption. Large acute abruption in a patient who admitted to cocaine abuse before onset of symptoms. Edge of placenta is detached (curved arrow) and there is a large retroplacental hematoma (arrow). Echogenic material in amniotic fluid (A) is consistent with an associated intraamniotic bleed. (P - placenta).

- 67% of abruptions > 20 weeks
  o Periplacental hematoma
    - Curvilinear hypoechoic blood seen in subchorionic space
    - Blood sometimes seen remote from placenta
  o **Raised edge of placenta seen in only 50% of cases**
- Retroplacental abruption
  o Blood in subchorionic space
  o **Placentomegaly** is most common acute finding
    - Isoechoic blood behind placenta
    - Concurrent bleed into placenta
  o **Power Doppler can help differentiate between blood and placenta**
- Preplacental abruption
  o Rare site
  o Hematoma on fetal surface of placenta
    - Subamniotic or subchorionic space
  o Hemorrhage may compress cord at origin
- **Intraamniotic blood**
  o Echogenic material in fluid, swallowed by fetus
  o May be seen with marginal and preplacental abruption

Imaging Recommendations
- Look for abruption first in patients presenting with pain and bleeding
- Stop exam and alert clinician if retroplacental abruption in viable fetus
- Power Doppler superior to color Doppler for differentiating hematoma from placenta
- **Estimate % of placenta detached**

Placental Abruption

Differential Diagnosis
Uterine Myoma
- Hypoechoic focus over which placenta may implant
- Myoma may affect outer contour of uterus
- Patient usually asymptomatic
- Color Doppler will show flow in myoma and rule out hematoma

Placenta Previa
- May clinically present like abruption (bleeding) but usually painless
- Low-lying placenta near or covering internal os
  - Sometimes with associated abruption

Pathology
General
- Etiology-Pathogenesis
  - Small vessel bleed into basal layer of decidua $\Rightarrow$ initiates abruption
  - Bleed splits decidua and spreads beneath placenta
  - Additional detachment occurs as hematoma spreads
- Epidemiology
  - 1% of all pregnancies
  - High-risk patients
    - **Previous placental abruption: 10 x increased risk**
    - Maternal hypertension
    - Cocaine use (related to hypertension)
    - Smoking
    - Increased parity
    - Trauma

Clinical Issues
Presentation
- Diagnosis is clinical
- Bleeding, pain, uterine contractions and tenderness
  - **80% present with bleeding +/- pain**
  - 20% with "trapped blood" and no bleeding
    - Higher risk for retroplacental abruption
    - **May present in preterm labor**
- **Most common in 3rd trimester but seen anytime after 20 weeks**

Treatment
- Depends on gestational age and maternal condition
- Self-limiting process in most cases: Expectant management
- Vaginal delivery possible in stable patients
- **Cesarean section** more common for symptomatic patients

Prognosis
- **Excellent if < 30% placenta detached**
- > 50% detachment associated with > 50% fetal death rate
- Acute sudden symptoms are associated with poor outcome
- Retroplacental hemorrhage associated with worst outcome

Selected References
1. Kramer MS et al: Etiologic determinants of abruptio placentae. Obstet Gynecol 89:221-9, 1997
2. Nyberg DA et al: Sonographic spectrum of placental abruption. AJR 148:161-4, 1987
3. McGahan JP et al: Sonographic spectrum of retroplacental hemorrhage. Radiology 142: 481-5, 1982

Placenta Accreta Spectrum

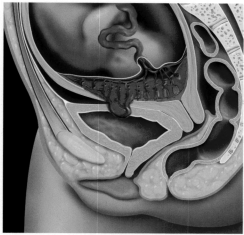

Placenta accreta spectrum. Drawing depicts sagittal section of maternal abdomen with placenta previa. Placental tissue breaches the anterior myometrium and invades the bladder. Decidua is absent at the site of abnormal placental invasion.

Key Facts
- Definition: Abnormal penetration of placental tissue beyond endometrial lining of uterus
- Classic imaging appearance
  - Loss of subplacental hypoechoic zone
  - "Abnormal" myometrial vascularity
- **Increased risk**
  - **Impaired ability to form decidua: Prior uterine surgery**
  - **Placenta previa**
- Spectrum of disease
  - **Accreta**: Placenta adherent to myometrium
  - **Increta**: Placenta invades myometrium
  - **Percreta**: Placenta invades through serosa +/- invades adjacent organs
- Maternal mortality: 7-10%; Fetal mortality: 9%

Imaging Findings
General Features
- Best imaging clue: **Loss of subplacental hypoechoic zone**
Ultrasound Findings
- Normal subplacental hypoechoic zone
  - Comprised of decidua basalis and myometrium
  - Should be present over entire placental surface
  - Normal bladder mucosa ⇒ echogenic reflector
- Findings associated with placental invasion
  - Placenta previa
  - Loss of subplacental hypoechoic zone
  - Loss of bladder reflector ⇒ percreta
  - Large vessels extending through myometrium +/- into bladder

Placenta Accreta Spectrum

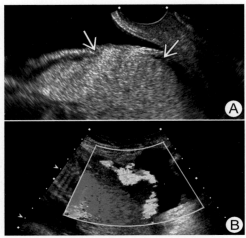

Placenta accreta spectrum. EV scans show loss of subplacental hypoechoic zone and the bladder mucosal reflector (arrows). TA color Doppler shows abnormal vessels extending from the placenta into the bladder. These are features of placenta percreta.

- o Anterior myometrium thinner than posterior
    - ▪ Best seen in early pregnancy
    - ▪ Scan EV if placenta previa

MR Findings
- • T2WI
    - o Loss of normal low-signal myometrium
    - o Extension of intermediate signal placental tissue beyond uterine margins
    - o Loss of fat planes between uterus/pelvic organs
- • Gadolinium (Gd) enhancement
    - o Gd crosses placenta
    - o Generally avoided in pregnancy
    - o Proponents argue risk/benefit ratio acceptable in life-threatening condition
- • MR Technique
    - o Pelvic coil centered on scar if prior C-section
    - o May require body coil for fundal/posterior placenta
    - o Bladder full to better evaluate for invasion
    - o Consider surgilube as vaginal contrast
    - o Axial, sagittal and coronal planes through placenta
    - o Fast scan techniques avoid fetal motion artifact

Imaging Recommendations
- • Serial scans: **Can progress from accreta to percreta**
- • High resolution linear transducer to assess abdominal wall, myometrial thickness
- • Endovaginal US best modality for previa/anterior placenta
- • MRI better for posterior placenta in at-risk patient
- • Preoperative MRI for extrauterine extent, cannot reliably diagnose accreta/increta

Placenta Accreta Spectrum

Differential Diagnosis
Uncomplicated Placenta Previa
- Intact subplacental hypoechoic zone

Pathology
General
- Abnormal placentation may predispose to bleeding diathesis
- Epidemiology
  - 1:70,000-93,000
  - **5% of patients with placenta previa**
  - **10% of patients with > 4 C-sections**
  - **67% of patients with placenta previa and > 4 C-sections**

Clinical Issues
Presentation
- Classical presentation: Uncontrollable hemorrhage in 3rd stage labor
- Increased awareness ⇒ active search in patients at risk
  - First trimester low sac position < 10 weeks ⇒ increase suspicion
  - Careful monitoring in 2nd and 3rd trimester allows preoperative planning
Treatment & Prognosis
- Risk of bleeding high even if spontaneous abortion or intrauterine demise
  - Uncontrollable hemorrhage described at D&C
- Consider hospitalization from 30 weeks
- Deliver at 34-35 weeks
  - Hemorrhagic complications increase markedly > 36 weeks
- Cesarean section with hysterectomy
- Consider delivery of infant only (placenta left in uterus)
  - Postoperative chemotherapy: Methotrexate
  - Postoperative embolization
  - Risk of postpartum hemorrhage (PPH)
  - Delayed hysterectomy for PPH theoretically safer
    - Reduction in uterine blood flow
- Consider pre-op placement arterial occlusion catheters
  - Anecdotal reports of effective control of bleeding
- Additional teams on standby for bladder/ureter/bowel invasion or injury
- **Significant risk maternal and fetal demise**
- **High morbidity**
  - 90% require transfusion
    - 40% ≥ 10 units
  - 28% postoperative infection
- MRI and US: Poor predictive value for all types (better for percreta)
  - Sensitivity MR 38%
  - Sensitivity US 33%
- **Manage for worst case scenario**

Selected References
1. Conrad JA et al: Placenta Percreta: Magnetic resonance imaging and temporary bilateral internal iliac artery balloon occlusion. Journal of Women's Imaging 4:139-44, 2002
2. Sonin AI: Nonoperative treatment of placental percreta: Value of MR imaging. AJR 177:1301-3, 2001
3. O'Brien J et al: The management of placenta percreta: Conservative and operative strategies. Am J Obstet Gynecol 175:1632-8, 1996

Placental Lakes

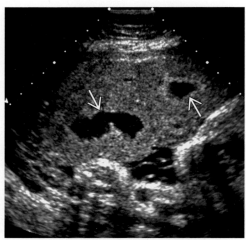

Placental lakes. Two hypoechoic masses are seen within the placenta (arrows). Subtle flow and variation in shape could be detected during real-time scanning.

Key Facts

- Synonyms: Intraplacental sonolucencies, venous lakes
- Definition: Enlargement of normal intervillous space with venous blood flow, hemorrhage, or fibrin
- Classic imaging appearance: **Focal lucent or hypoechoic areas** scattered within placenta
- **Commonly seen after 20 weeks** in normal pregnancies
- Increase in number with advancing pregnancy is normal
- May be **abnormal if diffuse or seen early in pregnancy**
  - Associated with
    - Elevated maternal serum alpha-fetoprotein (MSAFP)
    - First trimester bleeding
    - Placental insufficiency

Imaging Findings

General Features

- Best imaging clue: Prominent placental lucencies with or without blood flow, usually focal and scattered

Ultrasound Findings

- Occasional focal lucent or hypoechoic lesion
- May see **slow blood flow with standard gray-scale** imaging
  - Color Doppler may not show flow since it is very slow
- Lucencies often **change size and shape** during course of examination
- No flow in lucency suggests **fibrin deposition**
  - Not clinically significant unless diffuse involvement
  - Generally subchorionic
- Rarely **diffuse heterogeneous placenta** from multiple lesions
  - "Swiss cheese placenta"
    - Appearance may mimic trophoblastic change
  - Associated with
    - Elevated MSAFP

Placental Lakes

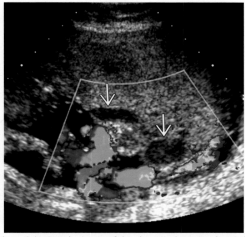

Placental lakes. Color Doppler image of the placenta shows two hypoechoic masses (arrows). Lack of perceptible flow rules out chorioangioma.

- Bleeding
  o Multiple fibrin deposits leads to a patchy appearance

Imaging Recommendations
- **Color Doppler** to evaluate vascularity
- Diffuse involvement or early finding
  o Pregnancy at risk for placental insufficiency
  o Follow up for growth and fluid
- Normal finding when lesions are sporadic and later in gestation
  o No follow-up necessary

Differential Diagnosis

Gestational Trophoblastic Neoplasia
- Partial mole
  o Triploid karyotype
  o Diffusely cystic placenta + living embryo or fetus
  o Fetus is abnormal with severe intra-uterine growth restriction (IUGR)
- Twin pregnancy with complete mole
  o Rare phenomenon with complete mole + normal twin
  o Two placentas: one cystic and one normal
    ▪ Normal placenta associated with normal fetus
    ▪ Cystic placenta, no fetus

Chorioangioma
- Benign placental tumor of small blood vessels
- Usually solitary circumscribed solid mass
- Hypo- or hyperechoic
- Often near umbilical cord origin site
- **Internal vascularity** on color Doppler
- Polyhydramnios may be present

Placental Hemorrhage
- Usually abruption
  o From edge (marginal) or retroplacental

Placental Lakes

- Symptomatic
  - o Bleeding
  - o Pain

Pathology
General
- General Path Comments
  - o Intraplacental hemorrhage may result from placental lakes and lead to intervillous thrombus and fibrin deposits
  - o Extensive fibrin deposit along basal plate (uterine side) may lead to maternal floor infarction
    - Risk of growth restriction and demise
    - Rare
- Etiology-Pathogenesis
  - o Enlarged normal intervillous spaces
  - o Intraplacental hemorrhage occurs with villous capillary breaks
  - o Intervillous thrombi lead to fibrin deposits
  - o Multiple or large lesions can lead to adjacent villous infarction
- Epidemiology
  - o Intervillous thrombi seen in 40% of term placentas
  - o Placental infarction seen in 25% of term placentas

Clinical Issues
Presentation
- Incidentally seen during ultrasound examination
- Elevated MSAFP
Natural History
- Common in third trimester
Treatment
- None necessary in vast majority of cases
- If associated placental insufficiency then early delivery may be necessary
Prognosis
- Usually excellent

Selected References
1. Harris RD et al: Sonography of the placenta with emphasis on pathologic correlation. Semin Ultrasound CT MRI 17:66-8, 1996
2. Bernstein IM et al: Elevated maternal serum alpha-fetoprotein: Association with placental sonolucencies, fetomaternal hemorrhage, vaginal bleeding, and pregnancy outcome in the absence of fetal anomalies. Obstet Gynecol 79:71-4, 1992
3. Spirt BA et al: Intervillous thrombosis: Sonographic and pathologic correlation. Radiology 147:197-200, 1983

Chorioangioma

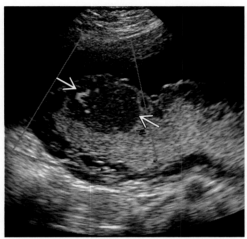

Small chorioangioma. Color Doppler ultrasound of the placenta shows a vascular, well-defined, hypoechoic mass on the fetal side of the placenta (arrows).

Key Facts
- Synonyms: Placental hemangioma, chorangioma
- Definition: Benign vascular placental tumor
- Classic imaging appearance: Solid, hypoechoic, vascular placental mass
- Typically incidental finding without sequelae
- **Polyhydramnios** common with large masses (etiology uncertain)
  - Proposed mechanism: Transudate from leaky tumor vessels
- May **rarely cause hydrops**
  - Secondary to **arteriovenous shunting**
- Most diagnosed in late 2nd and 3rd trimester
- Most common on **fetal side** of placenta, near cord insertion

Imaging Findings
General Features
- Best imaging clue: Will show **flow on color Doppler**
- **Greater arterial flow increases risk** of developing hydrops
- Usually solitary but may be multiple
- May be seen in umbilical cord
Ultrasound Findings
- Hypoechoic
- Well-defined
- More heterogeneous if internal hemorrhage
MR Findings
- T1WI: Isointense to placenta
  - May have high signal rim from hemorrhage
- T2WI: Heterogeneous high signal
Imaging Recommendations
- Measure mass
  - < 5 cm unlikely to have complications
  - > 5 cm evaluate for complications
    - Polyhydramnios

Chorioangioma

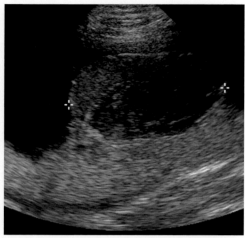

Large chorioangioma. Sonogram of the placenta shows a large, hypoechoic mass protruding into the amniotic cavity (cursors). Mild polyhydramnios was also present.

- Hydrops
- Intrauterine growth restriction
• Document vascularity
  o May be more important than size for predicting outcome
• Follow every 2-3 weeks for size and fetal assessment

Differential Diagnosis
Venous Lakes
• Look for subtle motion
  o Pooling venous blood
• Flow too slow to be seen with Doppler
Placental Hemorrhage
• No flow with Doppler
• Will evolve over time
Submucosal Fibroid
• On uterine side of placenta
Teratoma (Rare)
• Arises between amnion and chorion
• Irregular mass with calcification
Placental Metastases (Rare)
• Maternal
  o Melanoma
    - May metastasize to fetus
  o Breast
  o Lymphoma
• Fetal
  o Neuroblastoma
    - Large tumors
    - Hydrops usually present

Chorioangioma

Pathology
Genera1
- Associations
  - o Fetal hemangiomas
  - o Beckwith-Wiedemann syndrome
  - o Single umbilical artery
- Epidemiology
  - o 1% of placentas at delivery
    - Most too small to visualize by US

Microscopic Features
- 3 Types
  - o Angiomatous
    - Numerous blood vessels
    - Most likely to cause complications
  - o Cellular
    - Compacted endothelial cells
    - Few vessels
  - o Degenerated
    - Myxoid and hyaline deposition
    - Mass will become **more echogenic** and less vascular by US

Clinical Issues
Presentation
- Incidental finding
- Large masses
  - o Elevated alpha-fetoprotein
  - o Large-for-dates secondary to polyhydramnios

Treatment
- Generally none
- Amnioreduction for polyhydramnios
- Hydrops
  - o Transfusion for anemia
  - o Ligation or thermocoagulation of communicating vessels
    - Variable results

Prognosis
- Excellent without hydrops
- Poorer if hydrops present

Selected References
1. Jauniaux E et al: Color Doppler imaging in the diagnosis and management of chorioangiomas. Ultrasound Obstet Gynecol 15:463-7, 2000
2. Zoppini C et al: Varying clinical course of large placental chorioangiomas. Report of 3 cases. Fetal Diagn Ther 12:61-4, 1997
3. Bromley B et al: Solid masses on the fetal surface of the placenta: Differential diagnosis and clinical outcome. J Ultrasound Med 13:883-6, 1994

Hydatidiform Mole

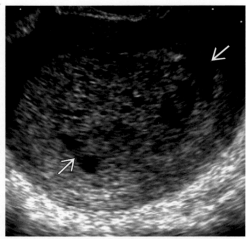

Hydatidiform mole. Uterus contains an echogenic mass with multiple cysts in this patient with elevated hCG levels and bleeding. Note associated crescent-shaped hemorrhage (arrows).

Key Facts
- Synonyms: Molar pregnancy, complete mole, classic mole
- Definition: Proliferative growth of trophoblastic tissue
- Classic imaging appearance: Enlarged uterus containing **echogenic mass with cysts and no fetal tissue**
- Most common type of gestational trophoblastic neoplasia
- Genetic make-up is 100% paternal
- **Usually diagnosed in first trimester**
- Associated with elevated human chorionic gonadotropin (hCG) levels
- Pathologic hallmark of diagnosis is **trophoblastic proliferation**
- Can develop into invasive mole or choriocarcinoma

Imaging Findings
General Features
- Best imaging clue: Echogenic mass, with cysts of various sizes, fills uterus
Ultrasound Findings
- **Variety of ultrasound findings in first trimester**
- Classic appearance
  - First trimester uterus filled with echogenic mass
  - High resolution ultrasound shows multiple small cysts
  - No embryo/fetus
  - Doppler ultrasound shows **low impedance, high velocity flow**
  - **Theca lutein cysts** in ovaries
    - 20-50% of cases, only when hCG levels are very high
    - Bilateral multiseptated ovarian cysts
- Mole **can look exactly like anembryonic pregnancy** (blighted ovum)
  - Gestational sac (GS) without normal internal structure
    - No yolk sac or abnormal yolk sac
    - GS mean measurement > 2 cm without living embryo
  - Diagnosis suspected clinically + elevated hCG levels

Hydatidiform Mole

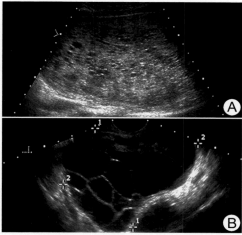

Hydatidiform mole. Early second trimester molar pregnancy. (A) Sagittal view of the uterus shows the endometrial cavity distended by an echogenic mass with multiple cysts. (B) Theca lutein cysts within a markedly enlarged left ovary (cursors) were also present.

- Second trimester mole
  - More severe findings
  - Uterus enlarged by cystic mass
  - Theca lutein cysts more likely
- **Coexistent mole and fetus**
  - Rare finding
  - Fetus is normal (unlike with triploidy/partial mole)
  - Mole represents trophoblastic neoplasia of **dizygotic twin**
- Complications detectable with ultrasound
  - **Hemorrhage**: Sonolucent areas within or adjacent to mass
  - **Invasive mole/Choriocarcinoma**
    - Up to 20% become invasive or metastatic (choriocarcinoma)
    - Suggested clinically by elevated hCG levels after treatment
    - Echogenic tissue invading myometrium may be seen

Imaging Recommendations
- When cystic change seen in early placenta, look at fetus
- With anembryonic pregnancy and cystic placenta, perform Doppler evaluation looking for high-velocity low-impedance flow

Differential Diagnosis
Hydropic Degeneration Of Placenta
- Seen with anembryonic pregnancy and embryonic demise
- Represents **hydropic change without trophoblastic proliferation**
- Can look identical to mole and pathologist must make diagnosis
- Doppler shows **low velocity, high impedance flow**
- Associated with low hCG levels
Placental Pseudomoles
- Mesenchymal dysplasia of placenta results in villus hydrops
- Often seen with pre-eclampsia and normal fetus

Hydatidiform Mole

- May be seen with placentomegaly and Beckwith-Wiedeman syndrome

Incomplete Mole/Partial Mole/Triploidy
- Cystic placenta
  - o Edematous villi with little trophoblastic proliferation
- Presence of **abnormal fetus** differentiates from classic mole
  - o Fetus with intrauterine growth restriction +/- multiple anomalies

Pathology
General
- Genetics
  - o **All nuclear DNA is paternal** in origin
  - o 46XX karyotype most common
    - ▪ **Egg with inactive or no nucleus** fertilized by sperm
    - ▪ Haploid sperm duplicates to diploid and cell division progresses
  - o 47XY karyotype uncommon
    - ▪ Egg with inactive or no nucleus fertilized by X and Y sperm
- Epidemiology
  - o 1:1,200 pregnancies in United States
  - o 1:100 pregnancies in Far East
  - o Increased risk with advanced maternal age
  - o 30x increased risk if prior mole

Microscopic Features
- Primary feature: Abnormal trophoblastic growth
- Swollen chorionic villi: Not a specific finding

Clinical Issues
Presentation
- **Hyperemesis**
- Symptoms of threatened abortion (bleeding, pain, closed cervix)
- Enlarged uterus for menstrual age
- **Elevated serum hCG levels**

Treatment
- Suction evacuation of uterus
- Curettage of endometrium to determine myometrial invasion
- Serial hCG levels

Prognosis
- Excellent
  - o **Cure rates of 90% even when invasive/choriocarcinoma**
- Invasive mole develops in 12-15%
- Metastatic choriocarcinoma develops in 5-8%

Selected References
1. Benson CB et al: Sonographic appearance of first trimester complete hydatidiform moles. Ultrasound Obstet Gynecol 16:188-91, 2000
2. Lazarus E et al: Sonographic appearance of early complete molar pregnancies. J Ultrasound Med 18:589-94, 1999
3. Jauniaux E et al: Early ultrasound diagnosis and follow up of molar pregnancies. Ultrasound Obstet Gynecol 9:17-21, 1999

Invasive Mole/Choriocarcinoma

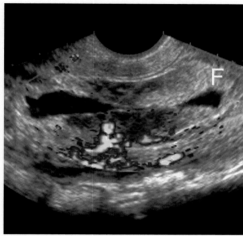

Invasive mole. Longitudinal image of a retropositioned uterus. Anterior myometrium is replaced by inhomogeneous vascular tissue. (F-fundus).

Key Facts
- Synonyms: Gestational trophoblastic disease (GTD), gestational trophoblastic neoplasia (GTN)
- Definition: Invasive tumor arising from abnormal proliferation of trophoblastic tissue
- Classic imaging appearance
  - Invasive mole
    - Focal areas increased echogenicity within myometrium
  - Choriocarcinoma
    - Widespread necrotic hemorrhagic metastatic deposits
- **GTN comprises a spectrum of conditions** with specific pathological and genetic features
  - Complete hydatidiform mole (CHM)
  - Partial mole (PM)
  - Invasive mole (IM)
  - Choriocarcinoma (CC)
  - Placental site trophoblastic tumor (PSTT)
  - Persistent GTN
- Associated with elevated human chorionic gonadotropin levels (hCG)
- Imaging helpful in diagnosis **GTD** as cause of vaginal bleeding
- **Imaging not decisive in managing non-metastatic GTD**
  - Integral role in staging and management metastatic disease

Imaging Findings
General Features
- Best imaging clue: Echogenic mass **invading myometrium**
Ultrasound Findings
- IM: Echogenic mass invading myometrium
  - Often vascular with high-velocity, low-impedance flow
  - Lesions may be occult at levels hCG < 700 mIU/ml
- Myometrial lesions may persist despite resolution of tumor

Invasive Mole/Choriocarcinoma

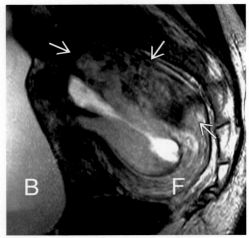

Invasive mole. Sagittal T2WI MRI. Uterus is retropositioned. The anterior myometrium is replaced by an inhomogeneous mass (arrows). Other scan planes showed invasion through the serosa. (F - fundus, B - bladder). The patient was successfully treated with methotrexate. Imaging and hCG returned to normal.

- CC primary tumor usually small (2-8 mm): Metastases dominant finding

<u>CT Findings</u>
- CECT: Useful for metastatic involvement brain, lungs, liver

<u>MR Findings</u>
- T2WI
  o Uterine enlargement
  o Disruption/complete loss zonal anatomy
  o Inhomogeneous intermediate signal myometrial masses
  o Flow voids: Highly vascular tumors
- Gadolinium enhancement: Depth myometrial invasion

<u>Other Modality Findings</u>
- Angiography supplanted by US and MR for staging
- Embolization useful to control bleeding

<u>Imaging Recommendations</u>
- **Remember sensitivity US/MR $\leq$ 70%**
- **Specificity even less**
- Use color Doppler: Vascularity IM < CC

Differential Diagnosis
<u>Retained Products of Conception (RPOC)</u>
- Low hCG levels
- RPOC in endometrial cavity, **never invades myometrium**

Pathology
<u>General</u>
- Genetics
  o 75% CC: Genomic imbalance of tumor suppressor genes/oncogenes
- Epidemiology
  o CC: 50% follow molar pregnancy

- 30% follow miscarriage
- 20% after normal pregnancy

Microscopic Features

- CC
  - Sheets of anaplastic cyto- and syncitiotrophoblast without chorionic villi
- IM
  - Extensive trophoblastic swelling and hyperplasia
  - Contains villi which penetrate myometrium or uterine vasculature

Staging or Grading Criteria

- **No universally accepted staging system**
  - Anatomic staging: International Federation of Gynecology and Obstetrics (**FIGO**)
    - Stage 1: Confined to uterine corpus (low risk for treatment failure)
    - Stage 2: Metastatic to pelvis/vagina
    - Stage 3: Pulmonary involvement
    - Stage 4: Distant metastases (require multi-agent chemotherapy)
  - Prognostic scoring: World Health Organization and National Institutes of Health (**WHO/NIH**)
    - Numerical scoring system using hCG levels, time since antecedent pregnancy, other clinical parameters
    - Main utility in FIGO Stage 2/3
    - WHO/NIH score >8 = "High risk": Treated with multiple agents
    - "Low-risk" Stage 2/3 treated with single-agent chemotherapy

Clinical Issues

Presentation

- **Elevated serum hCG level**
  - Remains elevated after pregnancy or treatment of CHM
- CC: Metastases ⇒ dyspnea, neurological symptoms, abdominal pain

Treatment

- Chemotherapy
- Monitor hCG levels
  - Weekly until normal x 3 then monthly x 6-12
- Surgery
  - For cure in selected group with no desire to preserve fertility
  - Bleeding: Uterine or from vaginal metastases
- Avoid pregnancy during follow up period
  - Elevated beta hCG from pregnancy complicates assessment of recurrent/persistent GTN

Prognosis

- Cure rates of 90%
- IM/CC highly chemosensitive
- Even high-risk metastatic disease
  - Complete remission in 75% with multi-agent chemotherapy
- Bleeding can be life threatening
  - **Use embolization:** May obviate emergent hysterectomy

Selected References
1. Li HW et al: Current understandings of the molecular genetics of gestational trophoblastic diseases. Placenta 23:20-31, 2002
2. Cohn D et al: Gestational trophoblastic disease: New standards for therapy. Current opinion in Oncology 12:492-6, 2000
3. Kohorn EI et al: Nonmetastatic gestational trophoblastic neoplasia. Role of ultrasonography and magnetic resonance imaging. J Reprod Med 43:14-20, 1998

Incompetent Cervix

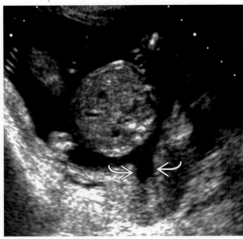

Incompetent cervix. Transabdominal ultrasound of the lower uterine segment shows a short cervix with internal os dilatation (arrows) in this asymptomatic woman at 20 weeks gestation.

Key Facts

- Definition: Preterm cervical effacement and/or cervical os dilatation
- Classic imaging appearance: Short cervical length (CL) for gestational age +/- internal os (IO) wedging/funneling before 35 weeks
- Best view of cervix is with **transvaginal ultrasound** (TVUS)
- **CL inversely correlates with risk of preterm birth**
- Earliest change in cervix involves internal cervical os
- 8-10% all births are preterm and account for > 70% neonatal deaths

Imaging Findings

General Features

- Best imaging clue: TVUS shows **CL < 25 mm at or before 24 wks and/ or IO funneling > 50% of CL**

Ultrasound Findings

- Cervical length (CL) findings
  - TVUS used to best measure full length accurately
  - Normal CL at 24 weeks
    - 34 +/- 8 mm nulliparous, 36 +/- 8 mm parous
  - Normal CL at 28 weeks
    - 33 +/- 8 mm nulliparous, 35 +/- 9 mm parous
  - < 25 mm at 24 weeks associated with 4 x increased risk for preterm birth
  - < 30 mm needs follow-up
- Cervical canal findings
  - IO Funneling: **Often first abnormality seen**
    - "Y-shaped" wedge of fluid and membranes
    - Funneling may extend into "V-shaped" wedge to external os (EO)
    - > 50% CL funneling associated with 79% preterm delivery
  - **Bulging membranes**
    - IO and EO open with protrusion of fluid and membranes

Incompetent Cervix

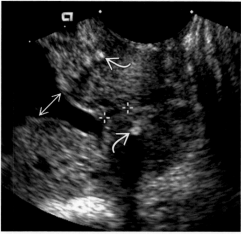

Incompetent cervix. Cerclage sutures are seen in anterior and posterior cervix (curved arrows). Internal os is distended (straight arrow) and calipers measure the distance between closed internal cervix and cerclage sutures. The functional (overall closed cervix) measured 15 mm in this case.

- o Hourglass membranes
    - ▪ Significant protrusion of fluid and membranes into upper vagina
- **Dynamic cervix**: Cervix appearance may change during exam
    - o Report worst appearance
        - ▪ Shortest CL
        - ▪ Widest IO funneling
    - o Dynamic change sometimes seen with **fundal pressure**
    - o When possible, examine cervix first (patient recently upright)
- Monitoring cervical **cerclage** (sutures placed in cervix)
    - o Sutures placed after 1st trimester or when early abnormal cervix seen
    - o Echogenic sutures seen in anterior and posterior lip (TVUS)
    - o Measure from point where cervix is closed to level of sutures
    - o Measure **closed portion of cervix = functional cervix**

Imaging Recommendations
- Transabdominal imaging of lower uterine segment routinely done
- TVUS for high risk patients
    - o **Prior preterm birth, prior cervix surgery, multiple gestation**
- **Transperineal ultrasound** when TVUS is contraindicated
    - o Ruptured membranes
    - o Known bulging membranes, hourglass membranes
    - o Active bleeding
- TVUS technique for CL measurement
    - o Insert probe carefully with direct visualization
    - o Find midline sagittal plane and angle for **best long-axis view**
    - o Pull probe back until external os seen well
    - o Measure from IO to EO 3 times
    - o If IO funneling seen, measure diameter and length
    - o Apply fundal pressure for 15 seconds and measure again
- Transperineal technique for CL measurement: More difficult

Incompetent Cervix

- o Elevate maternal hips to minimize artifact from bowel
- o Cover 3-5 MHz sector probe
- o Place probe on perineum, over labia minora
- o Use **collapsed vagina as acoustic window** to cervix
- o Same measurement technique as with TVUS

Differential Diagnosis
Overly Distended Bladder +/- Lower Uterine Contraction
- Can **mimic funneling as anterior and posterior uterus touch**
  - o Note associated thick myometrium
- Have patient void if bladder is full
- TVUS shows normal CL inferior to myometrium
- Tends to change/resolve with time

Nabothian Cyst
- Can mimic fluid in cervical canal
- TVUS shows cysts in anterior or posterior lip of cervix, not canal

Pathology
General
- Epidemiology
  - o **8-10% of all pregnancies result in preterm delivery**
  - o Preterm delivery cause of > 70% of neonatal deaths (normal babies)

Clinical Issues
Presentation
- Asymptomatic
- High risk patient
  - o Prior preterm delivery
  - o Multiple gestation
  - o Cone biopsy or other cervix surgery
- **Abnormal fetal fibronectin (fFN) test** result
  - o Speculum vaginal test looking at vaginal mucus for presence of fFN
  - o + test suggests disruption between chorion and decidual cavity
  - o + fFN and CL < 25 mm associated with 64% risk for preterm birth
  - o – fFN and CL< 25 mm associated with only 25% risk for preterm birth
  - o Can not do fFN if TVUS in last 24 h; when possible, do fFN first

Treatment
- Cerclage
  - o Many studies show no significant decrease in preterm birth
- Bed rest

Prognosis
- Depends on gestational age at delivery
- CL < 25 mm at 24 weeks associated with 4x increased risk for preterm birth
- Funneling > 50% CL associated with 79% increased risk for preterm birth

Selected References
1. Colombo DF et al: Cervical length and preterm labor. Clinic Obstet Gynecol 43:735-45, 2000
2. Wong G et al: Sonographic assessment of the cervix in pregnancy. Semin in Ultrasound CT and MR 19:370-80, 1998
3. Iams JD et al: The length of the cervix and the risk of spontaneous premature delivery. N Engl J Med 334:567-72, 1996

PocketRadiologist®

Obstetrics
Top 100 Diagnoses

TWINS

Dichorionic Diamniotic Twins

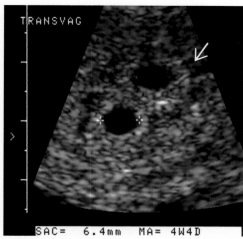

TRANSVAG

SAC= 6.4mm MA= 4W4D

Dichorionic diamniotic twins. EV US shows two gestational sacs surrounded by echogenic chorionic tissue. Cursors measure one sac. There is an echogenic chorionic reaction around the second sac (arrow). Dichorionicity conformed at < 5 weeks from LMP.

Key Facts
- Synonyms
  - Non-identical twins, fraternal twins: **Dizygotic** (DZ)
  - Identical twins: **Monozygotic** (MZ)
- Definition: Twins with separate chorionic sacs
- Classic imaging appearance: Two complete chorionic sacs seen in early first trimester
- Dichorionic (DC) twins
  - DZ in 2/3
  - MZ in 1/3
    - Division of zygote by 3rd day post conception
    - Chorion develops by 4th day
- MZ twins
  - DC 30%
  - Monochorionic diamniotic (MCDA) 60%
  - Monochorionic monoamniotic (MCMA) 10%

Imaging Findings
General Features
- Best imaging clue
  - **Thick echogenic chorion** completely surrounding each embryo
  - **Different gender** is most specific later sign
Ultrasound Findings
- Diagnosis easiest in early first trimester
  - Thick echogenic chorion surrounds sac completely
- Two yolk sacs
  - Specific sign of **diamniotic** gestation
  - DC twins must be diamniotic
- Fetal genders may be different in DZ
  - Will be same in MZ even when DC

Dichorionic Diamniotic Twins

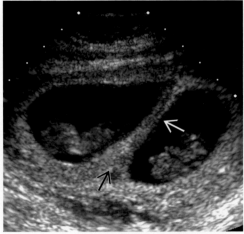

Dichorionic diamniotic twins. EV US shows two gestation sacs surrounded by echogenic chorionic tissue. The inter-twin membrane (white arrow) is thick. Chorionic tissue (black arrow) extends into the membrane. This gives rise to the "twin peak" sign.

- **Two placentas**
  - May be difficult to prove
    - Adjacent insertion sites
    - Placental fusion
    - Late presentation
- Thick inter-twin membrane
- **"Twin Peak" or Lambda sign**
  - Chorionic tissue extends into inter-twin membrane at placenta
  - Chorion is echogenic
  - Echogenic "triangle": Base on placental surface, apex in membrane

MR Findings
- May be of benefit to evaluate anomalies

Imaging Recommendations
- Look for anomalies
  - 2-3 x more common in twins than singletons
  - Monozygotic 50% > dizygotic
- Monitor growth
  - Growth restriction more common in multiples
- Watch for signs of crowding
  - Clubfoot
- Make sure amniotic fluid volume is symmetric
  - AFI difficult in twins
  - Use **single deepest pocket**
    - Sagittal scan plane
    - Probe **perpendicular to floor** not maternal abdomen

Differential Diagnosis
Monochorionic Diamniotic
- Must be same gender

Dichorionic Diamniotic Twins

- Single placental mass
- Thin inter-twin membrane

Pathology
General
- Genetics
  - **Dizygotic twinning increased with positive maternal history**
  - Paternal history not relevant
- Etiology-Pathogenesis
  - Embryology
    - Zygote divides within 3 days of conception
    - **Complete duplication of cell lines**
    - Formation of **separate chorion, amnion, embryo**
- Epidemiology
  - Twins 1:90 USA pregnancies
    - Accounts for 10% perinatal morbidity and mortality (MC > DC)
  - DZ
    - USA 7-11 per 1,000 births (geographic incidence varies)
    - Increased with maternal age and parity
    - Commoner with assisted reproduction
    - Positive maternal family history
  - MZ
    - 4 per 1,000 births
    - Independent of race/age/parity

Clinical Issues
Presentation
- Easily seen in first trimester endovaginal (EV) scans
- May present as
  - Size > dates
  - Hyperemesis
Treatment
- Monthly scans for growth and fluid volumes
- Increase frequency of monitoring if complications arise
Prognosis
- Maternal complications > singleton pregnancy
  - Preeclampsia/hypertension
  - Placenta previa/abruption
  - Hemorrhage: Pre/postpartum
- Higher incidence
  - Preterm delivery
    - **Twins 5 x singleton rate**
  - Intrauterine growth restriction
  - Anomalies
- Perinatal mortality reported 10%

Selected References
1. Shere DM: Adverse perinatal outcome of twin pregnancies according to chorionicity: Review of the literature. Am J Perinatol 18:23-37, 2001
2. Kiely JL: What is the population-based risk of preterm birth among twins and other multiples. Clin Obstet Gynecol 41:3-11, 1998
3. Benirshke K: The biology of the twinning process: How placentation influences outcome. Semin Perinatol 19:342-50, 1995

Monochorionic Diamniotic Twins

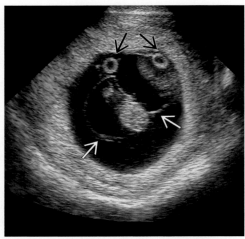

Monochorionic diamniotic twins. EV ultrasound at 6.8 weeks shows a single chorionic sac with two embryos, yolk sacs (black arrows) and amnions (white arrows). The amnions fuse to form the thin inter-twin membrane.

Key Facts
- Synonym: Identical twins
- Definition: Two fetuses resulting from division of single zygote between 4th and 8th day post conception
- Classic imaging appearance
  - Two fetuses
  - One placenta
  - Thin inter-twin membrane
- **Monozygotic (MZ) twinning**
- Monochorionic (MC) placentation ⇒ vascular connections between fetuses
- Specific complications may arise
  - Twin-twin transfusion syndrome (TTTS)
  - Twin reverse arterial perfusion syndrome (TRAP)
  - Twin embolization syndrome (TES)

Imaging Findings
General Features
- Best imaging clue: **Thin inter-twin membrane**
  - Subjective
  - No specific measurement
  - **Difficult in 3rd trimester**: All membranes look thin
Ultrasound Findings
- **Two yolk sacs in first trimester**
- Single placental mass
- Thin inter-twin membrane
- Twins must be same gender
- No "twin peak" (lambda sign)
MR Findings
- May be of benefit to evaluate anomalies
- Pre/post fetal intervention

Monochorionic Diamniotic Twins

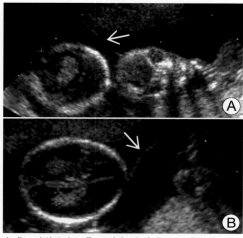

Monochorionic diamniotic twins. Transabdominal ultrasounds in the second trimester showing two examples of thin inter-twin membrane (white arrows).

Imaging Recommendations
- Look for anomalies: Increased incidence in all twins
- Attempt to identify **placental cord insertion** sites
  - Increased incidence of marginal cord insertion
    - Unequal placental sharing
    - Increased risk for discordant growth
  - Increased incidence of vasa previa
    - Fetal vessels crossing internal os
    - Labor ⇒ vessels tear ⇒ fetal exsanguination
- Monitor growth: Growth restriction more common in multiples
- **Discordant growth**
  - > 15-20% difference is estimated fetal weight (EFW)
  - > 20 mm difference in abdominal circumference (AC)
  - By convention only used when one twin has intra-uterine growth restriction (IUGR)
  - If neither twin IUGR, use asymmetric/disparate growth
- Check for **symmetric amniotic fluid volume**
  - Asymmetric distribution important sign of TTTS
  - If discordant growth, smaller twin may have oligohydramnios
  - Oligohydramnios in one sac may ⇒ anomaly
- Look for specific complications of monochorionic twinning
  - TTTS/TRAP/TES

Differential Diagnosis
Dichorionic Diamniotic
- **Fused placentas may appear as one**
- Twin peak sign present
- Inter-twin membrane thicker
- Inter-twin membrane composed of four layers
  - High resolution probe may show multiple layers
  - Most useful in late presentation

Monochorionic Diamniotic Twins

- Fetal **gender** may differ in dizygotic DC twinning

Monochorionic Monoamniotic
- No inter-twin membrane
- Cord entanglement may occur

Pathology
General
- TTTS: See "Twin-Twin Transfusion"
- TRAP: See "Twin Reversed Arterial Perfusion"
- Twin embolization syndrome: Two theories
  o Older hypothesis
    - Twin demise ⇒ tissue necrosis
    - Embolization of live twin
  o Current theory
    - Twin demise ⇒ loss of peripheral resistance
    - MC placentation ⇒ vascular anastomoses between twins
    - Abrupt drop in peripheral resistance ⇒ hypotension in live twin
    - Same end result: "Hypoperfusion" lesions of brain/kidneys
    - Porencephaly/periventricular leukomalacia/renal infarction
- Genetics
  o MZ twinning independent of race/family history
- Etiology-Pathogenesis
  o Embryology
    - Inner cell mass of blastocyst splits between **4th and 8th** day post conception
    - Chorion already formed
    - Division results in formation of two amnions and two embryos
    - Division after 8th day ⇒ monochorionic monoamniotic twins
- Epidemiology
  o 60% of monozygotic twins
  o MZ twins 4:1,000 births
  o Chemically induced pregnancies mostly DZ
    - But **MZ twinning rate is 8 x** general population rate

Clinical Issues
Presentation
- Best seen on first trimester endovaginal (EV) scans
Treatment & Prognosis
- Monthly scans for growth and fluid
- Careful watch for complications
  o See "Twin-Twin Transfusion"
  o See "Twin Reversed Arterial Perfusion"
- **MC twins 3-5 x DC twins incidence perinatal morbidity and mortality**
- Earlier diagnosis, aggressive monitoring, early hospitalization have improved outcome

Selected References
1. Gaziano AP et al: Diamniotic monochorionic twin gestations: An overview. J Matern Fetal Med 8:89-96, 2000
2. Al-Kouatly HB et al: Twin Pregnancy. Curr Opin Obstet Gynecol 11:125-9, 1999
3. Monteagudo A et al: Early and simple determination of chorionic and amniotic type in multifetal gestations in the first fourteen weeks by high-frequency transvaginal ultrasonography. Am J Obstet Gynecol 170:824-9, 1994

Monochorionic Monoamniotic Twins

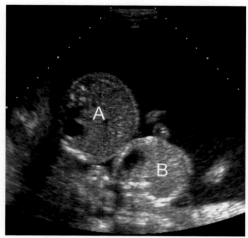

Monochorionic monoamniotic twins. Second trimester ultrasound shows twins in a single sac with no inter-twin membrane. Both twins are imaged transversely through the abdomen. Twin B is smaller.

Key Facts
- Definition: Twin fetuses occupying single amniotic sac
- Classic imaging appearance: Twins with no inter-twin membrane
- Monochorionic twinning
  - Single placental mass
  - Twins same sex
- Division of zygote occurs after 8th post conception day
  - First 3 days ⇒ dichorionic diamniotic twins
  - Between 4th and 8th days ⇒ monochorionic diamniotic twins
  - After 13th day ⇒ conjoined twins
- Perinatal mortality 54%

Imaging Findings
General Features
- Best imaging clue: No inter-twin membrane
Ultrasound Findings
- Single yolk sac in first trimester
- Single placental mass
- Same gender
- No inter-twin membrane
- **Umbilical cord entanglement**
  - Cord appears to branch
  - Mass of vessels with different fetal heart rates
  - Side by side placental insertion may increase risk
- Umbilical Artery (UA) Doppler
  - End systolic notch in UA abnormal
  - May reflect hemodynamic alterations in vessels narrowed by knot
MR Findings
- Use to evaluate brain injury
- Clarify anomalies if present

Monochorionic Monoamniotic Twins

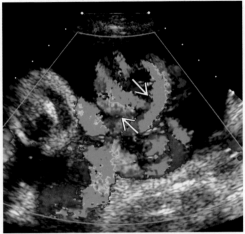

Monochorionic monoamniotic twins. Color Doppler shows cord entanglement with apparent branching of the umbilical cord (arrows).

Imaging Recommendations
- **Number yolk sacs = number amnions** but yolk sac easier to see
  - If only one yolk sac, early follow-up, occasionally second sac development delayed
- Fetal gender: If different => dizygotic twins
- Assess umbilical cord
  - Insertion site
  - Entanglement
  - Spectral analysis
- Careful search for anomalies

Differential Diagnosis
Conjoined Twins
- Contiguous skin covering at same anatomic plane
- Cords may be fused but do not appear knotted
Diamniotic Twins With "Absent" Inter-Twin Membrane
- Twin-twin transfusion syndrome (TTTS)
  - Donor twin in fixed position = "stuck" twin
  - Shunt twin larger, polyhydramnios +/ - hydrops
- Twin demise
  - Anhydramnios in sac of deceased twin
  - Membrane closely applied to dead fetus therefore not seen
  - Dead co-twin in fixed position with no cardiac activity
- Twin anomaly
  - Renal agenesis/sirenomelia in one twin
- Premature rupture of membranes
  - Anhydramnios around presenting twin
- Intrauterine membrane rupture
  - Failure to see membrane after earlier documentation
  - Trauma/infection
  - Developmentally abnormal membrane

Monochorionic Monoamniotic Twins

Pathology

General
- Embryology
  - Embryo splits after 8th post conception day
  - Cells already committed to chorion and amnion
  - 2 embryos within single amniotic sac
- Epidemiology
  - < 1% of monozygotic twinning
  - F>M
  - Rare event ⇒ true incidence uncertain

Clinical Issues

Presentation
- Cord entanglement described as early as 10 weeks
  - Successful outcome reported despite pathological confirmation of cord knot

Treatment
- Monthly scans to assess
  - Growth
  - Polyhydramnios
  - TTTS
- Intensive monitoring
  - Daily nonstress testing (NST) from 26 weeks
  - Increasing frequency of decelerations may herald serious cord compression
  - Continuous heart monitoring if variable decelerations increase in frequency or severity
  - Biophysical profile for nonreactive NST
- Safety of expectant management beyond 34 weeks gestation unproven
  - Elective delivery at 34 weeks after maternal corticosteroid administration or
  - Deliver at lung maturity
- Cesarean section: Preferred but successful vaginal deliveries have occurred

Prognosis
- 54% perinatal mortality rate
  - Prematurity
  - Growth restriction
  - Anomalies
  - Cord accidents
  - Vascular anastomoses
  - Twin-twin transfusion
- Old data suggested double (both twins) survival rare
- Modern management ⇒ double survival more likely

Selected References
1. Sherer DM et al: Diagnosis of umbilical cord entanglement of monoamniotic twins by first trimester color Doppler imaging. J Ultrasound Med 21:1307-9, 2002
2. Su LL: Monoamniotic twins: Diagnosis and management. Acta Obstet Gynecol Scand 81:995-1000, 2002
3. Seibre NJ et al: First trimester diagnosis of monoamniotic twin pregnancies. Ultrasound Obstet Gynecol 16:223-5, 2000

Conjoined Twins

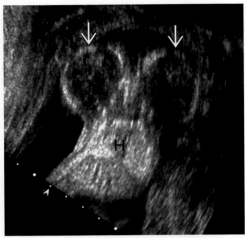

Conjoined twins. Ultrasound image of dicephalus conjoined twins. There are two cranial vaults (arrows) but neither twin had a separate face. Echogenic lungs are seen above an intact diaphragm and there is a single heart (H). The mother requested termination of pregnancy.

Key Facts
- Definition: Fetal fusion of variable degree
- Classic imaging appearance: Twins with contiguous skin covering at same anatomic plane
- Monochorionic twinning
- Nomenclature
  o Site of fusion + suffix "pagus"
    - Thoracopagus: Fused at chest
    - Omphalopagus: Fused xiphoid to umbilicus
    - Thoraco-omphalopagus: Extensive chest and abdominal fusion
  o "Di" + completely separate parts
    - Dicephalus: Conglomerate mass with two identifiable heads

Imaging Findings
General Features
- Best imaging clue: Contiguous skin covering between fetuses
Ultrasound Findings
- Fetuses inseparable
- Discordant presentation does not exclude diagnosis
  o Fused tissue may be pliable, relative position not always constant
- No inter-twin membrane
- Single placental mass
- Often hyperextension of cervical spines
- Unusual limb positioning
- Fused umbilical cord, 2 to 7 vessels
- Fetal echocardiography
  o Better acoustic access in utero than post delivery
  o Thoracopagus share pericardium in 90%, heart in 75%
  o Omphalopagus share liver in 80%, 30% congenital heart disease (CHD)

Conjoined Twins

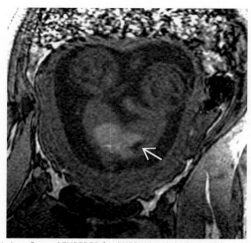

Conjoined twins. Coronal FMPSPGR fetal MRI. Liver is high signal (arrow). These are thoraco-omphalopagus twins. The twin on the maternal right has the majority of the liver. These twins were delivered at 34 weeks. Separation will be attempted when they are larger and stronger.

CT Findings
- Occasionally used for confirmation

MR Findings
- Pre-surgical planning
  - No sedation
  - Fetuses stable on placental support
- Degree shared organs particularly brain
  - SSFSE
    - Excellent for brain/renal/chest detail
  - FMPSPGR
    - Liver high signal
    - Meconium-filled bowel high signal

Imaging Recommendations
- Look for different heart rates: Proves hearts not shared/fused
- Use color Doppler in craniopagus
  - Partial: Brains separate, cranium shared
  - Complete: Shared brain substances precludes separation
  - If separated by arachnoid only, separation determined by venous sinuses
- 3D may help parents to understand complex anatomy
- 2D/Doppler more definitive specific information on shared organs
- Fetal MRI

Differential Diagnosis
Twin Reverse Arterial Perfusion (TRAP)
- One fetus with cranial/upper body malformation
- Abnormal fetus perfused by co-twin
  - Flow in umbilical artery **toward** abnormal fetus
- Inter-twin membrane present if diamniotic

Conjoined Twins

Monoamniotic Twins
- No inter-twin membrane
- Fetuses in same sac but no contiguous skin covering
- Two cords
  o May have common origin
  o Cord knot: Vessels appear branched

Pathology
General
- Embryology-Anatomy
  o Incomplete cleavage embryonic disc after 13th day post-conception
- Epidemiology
  o 1:50,000 to 1:100,000 births
  o 70% female

Clinical Issues
Presentation
- Can be diagnosed in first trimester
Treatment
- Offer termination
- If pregnancy continues
  o Fetal echocardiogram
  o Deliver at tertiary center
- Cesarean section required
  o Mechanical obstruction precludes vaginal delivery
  o In third trimester requires "classical" uterine incision
    ▪ Increased maternal morbidity
    ▪ Precludes future vaginal delivery
- Not indication for early deliver
  o Morbidity and mortality increase with low birth weight
- Separation if feasible
  o Delayed separation preferred
  o Emergent separation required for potentially lethal situation
    ▪ One twin with rudimentary heart
Prognosis
- Majority deliver preterm
- 40% stillborn
- 75% die within first 24 hrs of life
- If live to separation
  o 50% survive neonatal separation
  o 90% survive separation at > 4 months of age
    ▪ Bigger, stronger baby
    ▪ Placement of skin expanders prior to definitive surgery
- Long term morbidity from associated defects, unequal sharing of limbs and major organs

Selected References
1. Bonilla-Musolles F et al: Two-dimensional and three-dimensional sonography of conjoined twins. J Clin Ultrasound 30:68-75, 2002
2. Mackenzie TC et al: The natural history of prenatally diagnosed conjoined twins. J Pediatr Surg 37:303-9, 2002
3. Spielman AL et al: MRI of conjoined twins illustrating advances in fetal imaging. J Comput Assist Tomogr 25:88-90, 2001

Twin-Twin Transfusion Syndrome

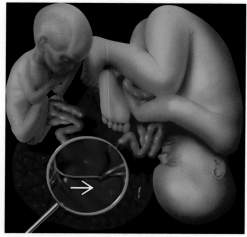

Twin-twin transfusion syndrome. Illustration depicts discordant twins. Larger recipient twin, smaller donor twin. Abnormal arteriovenous communications (arrow) are seen on the placental surface. Arterial de-oygenated blood from donor mixes with venous oxygenated blood returning to recipient .

Key Facts
- Synonym: Twin oligohydramnios polyhydramnios sequence (TOPS)
- Definition: Monochorionic twinning with **artery-to-vein anastomoses** in placenta allowing donor twin to partly perfuse recipient twin
- Classic imaging appearance
  - Monochorionic (MC) twins
  - Discordant growth
  - Smaller fetus: Oligohydramnios
  - Larger fetus: Polyhydramnios

Imaging Findings
General Features
- Best imaging clue: Discordant monochorionic twins with asymmetric fluid distribution
Ultrasound Findings
- Single placental mass
- Twins same gender
- Asymmetric distribution of fluid about inter-twin membrane
  - Polyhydramnios defined as deepest pocket ≥ 8 cm
  - Oligohydramnios defined as deepest pocket ≤ 2 cm
- **"Stuck twin"** when almost no fluid seen about smaller twin
- Twins usually discordant but lesser degrees of growth discrepancy do not exclude diagnosis
MR Findings
- Confirm normal brain structure prior to intervention
- Follow for adverse sequelae of laser coagulation of shunt vessels
  - Intracranial hemorrhage/deep white matter injury
Imaging Recommendations
- Stage twin-twin transfusion syndrome (TTTS)
  - Stage 1: Donor bladder visible, normal Doppler

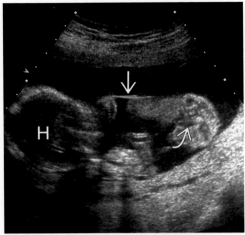

Twin-twin transfusion syndrome. Ultrasound demonstrating "stuck twin" appearance, inter-twin membrane is seen only where it is stretched between upper & lower extremities (arrow). The bladder is empty indicating renal hypoperfusion in donor, (curved arrow). (H – head).

- o Stage 2: Donor bladder empty, normal Doppler
- o Stage 3: Donor bladder empty, abnormal Doppler
- o Stage 4: Hydrops
- o Stage 5: Demise of one or both
- Criteria for abnormal Doppler
- o Umbilical artery: Absent or reversed end diastolic flow
- o Umbilical vein: Pulsatile flow
- o Ductus venosus: Reversed flow
- Fetal echocardiography
- o Congenital heart disease (CHD) more prevalent in TTTS than in uncomplicated monochorionic diamniotic (MCDA) pregnancies
  - ▪ MCDA: TTTS = 2.3%:6.9%
  - ▪ Recipient twin: 11.9%
- o Functional problems relating to TTTS in recipient
  - ▪ Biventricular hypertrophy
  - ▪ Impaired ventricular function
  - ▪ Tricuspid regurgitation
  - ▪ Cardiac enlargement
- o Donor twins without CHD have normal fetal echo

Differential Diagnosis
Premature Rupture of Membranes
- Ask the patient
Twin Demise
- Absent cardiac activity in oligohydramnios sac
Anomalous Twin
- Renal agenesis/sirenomelia in one twin

Twin-Twin Transfusion Syndrome

Pathology
General
- Often marginal insertion of donor cord
- Etiology-Pathogenesis
  - ≥ 1 Arteriovenous anastomoses within MC placenta
    - Unidirectional flow: Donor to recipient
    - Transfusion occurs within placental cotyledon
    - Vessels enter and leave cotyledon via common foramen
    - "Nose-to-nose" appearance different to normal paired vessels
    - Readily seen at fetoscopy
    - Abnormal connection can be identified sonographically to guide selective laser coagulation
  - +/- Absence of bidirectional (to and from both fetuses) arterioarterial anastomoses
    - Direct lumenal contact on placental surface
    - Found in most MC placentas
    - Generally no net shunt
    - May be protective against TTTS: Compensate for unbalanced donor ⇒ recipient shunt in AV anastomosis
- Epidemiology
  - Complicates 10-20% of monochorionic pregnancies

Clinical Issues
Presentation
- Can be detected in first trimester
- Often presents later
Treatment
- UK approach
  - Serial amnioreduction/septostomy for early stage disease
  - Laser coagulation of shunt vessels reserved for more severe cases
    - Risk procedure-related fetal loss
- USA: Multi-center study currently enrolling patients to determine
  - If fetoscopic laser coagulation ⇒ improved survival of twins with severe TTTS vs serial amnioreduction
  - If fetoscopic laser coagulation ⇒ improved cardiac, neurological and developmental outcomes of twins with severe TTTS vs. serial amnioreduction
Prognosis
- Progressive disorder > 90% mortality if untreated
- Stage at presentation does not correlate with outcome
- Change of stage during treatment alters prognosis
  - Decreased stage: 94% survival
  - Increased stage: 27% mortality
- Morbidity common in survivors
  - Neurological: 5-23% especially if co-twin demise
  - Cardiac: Most functional changes resolve within 6 months

Selected References
1. Wee LY et al: The twin-twin transfusion syndromes. Semin Neonatol 7:187-202, 2002
2. Karatza AA et al: Influence of twin-twin transfusion syndrome on fetal cardiovascular structure. Heart 19:550-5, 2002
3. Feldstein V et al: Twin-twin transfusion syndrome: The "select" procedure. Fetal Diagn Ther 15:257-61, 2000

Twin Reversed Arterial Perfusion

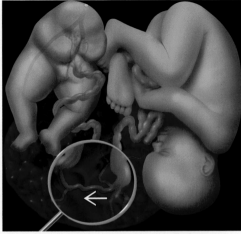

Twin reversed arterial perfusion. Image depicts normal twin perfusing abnormal co-twin via artery (de-oxygenated blood) to artery placental anastomosis (arrow). Abnormal circulation impairs development of the heart, head and torso.

Key Facts
- Synonyms: Acardiac monster, cardiac regression sequence
- Definition
  - Acardiac twin perfused by deoxygenated blood from "pump" twin
  - Blood enters embryo via umbilical artery = reversed perfusion
    - Normal perfusion: Oxygenated blood from placenta via umbilical vein
- Classic imaging appearance
  - Single placental mass
  - One normal twin
  - One twin with no cardiac activity and amorphous upper torso
- Monochorionic twinning
  - Can occur in mono or diamniotic types
- Placental artery-to-artery anastomosis

Imaging Findings
General Features
- Best imaging clue: Flow in umbilical artery of abnormal twin is **toward fetus**
Ultrasound Findings
- Single umbilical artery in 66% acardiac twins
- Pump twin structurally normal but at risk for hydrops
- Polyhydramnios
  - Strong correlation with presence of renal tissue in acardiac twin
- Doppler shunt vessels
  - Artery to artery pulsatile flow
  - Vein to vein non pulsatile flow in opposite direction
  - Identification assists laser coagulation

Twin Reversed Arterial Perfusion

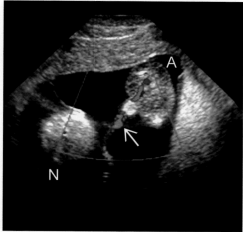

Twin reversed arterial perfusion. Ultrasound image shows arterial flow (arrow) in the umbilical artery going towards the abnormal (A) acardiac fetus. Normal UA flow is away from the fetus. This flow could be traced back to the normal (N) twin.

MR Findings
- SSFSE
  - Confirm normal brain structure prior to intervention
  - Follow for adverse sequela of laser coagulation of shunt vessels

Imaging Recommendations
- Monitor growth
- Estimated fetal weight (EFW) acardiac/pump > 50%
  - Increased risk polyhydramnios and pre-term labor

Differential Diagnosis

Twin Demise
- Should be anhydramnios in sac of dead twin if diamniotic
- No flow in dead twin cord
- Demise may be secondary to anomalies but should be identifiable cranial and upper body structures

Conjoined Twins
- No inter-twin membrane
- Contiguous external skin contour

Pathology

General
- Genetics
  - Not hereditary: No recurrence risk
- Epidemiology
  - 1% monochorionic pregnancies
  - 1:35,000 births
- Etiology-Pathogenesis: Two theories
  - Primary defect in cardiac embryogenesis
    - Reverse perfusion allows continued development

Twin Reversed Arterial Perfusion

- o Reverse perfusion from artery-to-artery placental anastomoses
    - ▪ Secondary cardiac/upper body maldevelopment
    - ▪ Better explanation of anatomic findings

Gross Pathologic, Surgical Features
- Broad spectrum of anomalies: 4 subtypes described
    - o Acardius acephalus: Commonest
        - ▪ Well-developed pelvis, lower extremities
    - o Acardius anceps: Rudimentary cranial structures
    - o Acardius amorphous: No identifiable human features
    - o Acardius acormus: Rarest
        - ▪ Head develops without body
- Pseudoacardius: Malformed twin with remnants of cardiac structures

Clinical Issues

Presentation
- Described in first trimester
- Case reports of twins with cardiac activity in both
    - o Subsequent loss of cardiac activity in one fetus
    - o Reverse perfusion allows continued but abnormal growth

Natural History
- Spontaneous closure of shunt vessels reported

Treatment
- Offer termination
- Offer karyotype: 33% abnormal
- Conservative nonintervention
- Intervention
    - o Endoscopic laser coagulation of shunt vessels < 24 weeks
    - o Ligation of acardiac umbilical cord after 24 weeks
        - ▪ Endoscopic or sonographic guidance
    - o Other reported treatments
        - ▪ Hysterotomy with selective delivery of acardiac twin
        - ▪ US-guided embolization of acardiac umbilical artery

Prognosis
- Recipient twin anomalies lethal
- Pump twin mortality 50-75%: Increased with
    - o Hydrops in pump twin
    - o Polyhydramnios
    - o Preterm delivery
    - o Developed arms, ears, kidneys in acardiac twin
- Pump twin mortality reduced to 13.6% with fetal surgery
    - o 22 cases total culled from literature review

Selected References
1. Driggers RW et al: Pathogenesis of acardiac twinning: clues from an almost acardiac twin. Fetal Diagn Ther 17:185-7, 2002
2. Coulam CB et al: First trimester diagnosis of acardiac twins. Early Pregnancy 4:261-70, 2000
3. Arias F et al: Treatment of acardiac twinning. Obstet Gynecol 91:818-21, 1998

PocketRadiologist®
Obstetrics
Top 100 Diagnoses

CHROMOSOMES

Trisomy 21

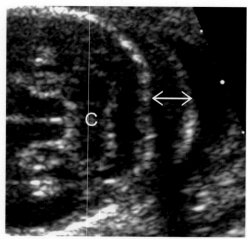

Trisomy 21. Increased nuchal fold thickness in this second trimester fetus with trisomy 21 (arrow). Measurement is taken on an axial image through posterior fossa from outer table of skull to skin/amniotic fluid interface. Care is taken not to angle coronally since nuchal fold may appear falsely increased. (C-cerebellum).

Key Facts
- Synonym: Down syndrome
- Definition: Autosomal trisomy of chromosome 21
- Classic imaging appearance: First trimester increased **nuchal translucency** or second trimester fetus with **minor markers** for trisomy 21 (T21) +/- major anomalies
- **Increased nuchal thickness is most sensitive 2nd trimester marker**
- 50-70% T21 fetuses can be identified with ultrasound in 2nd trimester
  - < 20% have major anomalies thus minor markers are important
- 60-70% detection rates with maternal serum biochemistry results
  - 5% false positive rate
- Most common chromosome abnormality resulting in live birth
- Associated with **advanced maternal age** (> 35 years at time of delivery)

Imaging Findings
<u>General Features</u>
- Best imaging clue: First trimester increased nuchal lucency or 2nd trimester fetus with several minor markers for T21
<u>Ultrasound Findings</u>
- Major anomalies (< 20%)
  - Cardiac defects (25%)
    - **Atrioventricular septal defect** (endocardial cushion defect)
    - Ventriculoseptal defect
    - Tetralogy of Fallot
  - Gastrointestinal anomalies (8%)
    - **Duodenal atresia**: Rarely detectable before 20 wks
    - Esophageal atresia: Polyhydramnios in 3rd trimester
    - Omphalocele

Trisomy 21

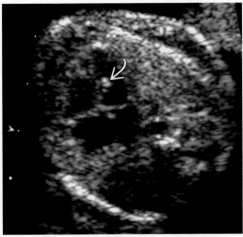

Trisomy 21. Echogenic cardiac focus (as bright as bone) in the left ventricle (arrow). This is a minor marker for trisomy 21 and caused by mineralization of papillary musculature. This fetus with trisomy 21 also had echogenic bowel and renal pelviectasis.

- o Central nervous system anomalies (4%)
  - ▪ Ventriculomegaly: Most common
- **Minor markers in 2nd trimester** (15-21 wks): 1 or more in 50-70%
  - o Nuchal thickening
    - ▪ Skin measures **> 5 mm** on routine posterior fossa view
    - ▪ Measurement taken from skull outer table to skin/fluid interface
    - ▪ **Most sensitive and specific single marker**, false + rate < 1%
    - ▪ Likelihood ratio= 11 (11 times more likely than apriori risk for T21)
  - o Short femur length (FL) and humerus length (HL)
    - ▪ Long bone measurements compared to biparietal diameter (BPD)
    - ▪ Expected FL = -9.3 + 0.90 (BPD)
    - ▪ Expected HL = -7.9 + 0.84 (BPD)
    - ▪ Abnormal ratio = measure: expected FL $\leq$ 0.91 and HL $\leq$ 0.90
    - ▪ Likelihood ratio = 5.1 for short humerus, 1.5 for short femur
  - o Echogenic bowel
    - ▪ Focal echogenic bowel as bright as bone (grade 2)
    - ▪ Likelihood ratio = 6.7
  - o Intracardiac echogenic focus (IEF)
    - ▪ Bright dot, as echogenic as bone, in left or right ventricle of heart
    - ▪ 3-4% of normal fetuses and more common in Asian population
    - ▪ Multiple or bilateral IEF increases risk
    - ▪ Likelihood ratio: 1.8
  - o Renal pelviectasis
    - ▪ Fluid filled renal pelvis measured in anterior-posterior dimension
    - ▪ > 3 mm
    - ▪ 3% of normal fetuses
    - ▪ Likelihood ratio: 1.6
  - o Other minor markers seen with T21

Trisomy 21

- 5th finger clinodactyly: Hypoplastic mid-phalanx, distal finger curves inward
- Sandal gap foot: Wide gap between 1st and 2nd toes

Imaging Recommendations
- Look for additional minor markers when appropriate
- **Routine nuchal fold measurements** in all fetuses between 15-22 wks

Differential Diagnosis
Isolated Minor Markers
- All minor markers, in isolation, are more common in normal fetuses
- Presence of multiple minor markers raises more suspicion

Pathology
General
- Genetics
  o Autosomal trisomy of chromosome 21
- Epidemiology
  o **1:504** 2nd trimester pregnancies
  o **Age-related risk** of 1:1,176 at 20 yrs, 1:274 at 35 yrs, 1:42 at 42 yrs

Staging or Grading Criteria
- Genetic scan, looking for minor markers, can be used to change patient's baseline (apriori) risk for T21 and help decide about amniocentesis
- **Scoring index system**: Amniocentesis when additive score is $\geq$ 2
  o Increased nuchal thickness = 2
  o Major anomalies = 2
  o Each minor marker = 1

Clinical Issues
Presentation
- Ultrasound findings during routine obstetrical exam in low-risk patient
- Genetic sonogram in high-risk patient
- **Abnormal maternal serum quadruple test screen** result
  o Low alpha-fetoprotein (AFP)
  o High human chorionic gonadotropin protein (hCG)
  o Low estriol
  o High inhibin A protein

Prognosis
- Mean survival to age 20 (prognosis related to associated anomalies)
- Mental retardation: Mean IQ of 50-60
- 20-fold increased risk for acute leukemia
- Hearing loss in 90%

Selected References
1. Bromley B et al: The genetic sonogram: A method of risk assessment for Down syndrome in the second trimester. J Ultrasound Med 21:1087-96, 2002
2. Nyberg DA et al: Age-adjusted ultrasound risk assessment for fetal Down syndrome during the second trimester: Description of the method and analysis of 142 cases. Ultrasound Obstet Gynecol 12:8-14, 1998
3. Benacerraf BR et al: Sonographic scoring index for prenatal detection of chromosomal abnormalities. J Ultrasound Med 11:449-58, 1992

Trisomy 18

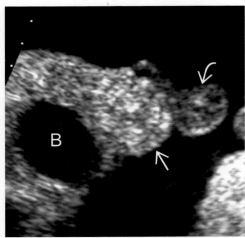

Trisomy 18. Ultrasound image shows an omphalocele containing only bowel (arrow). Note bowel is not free floating (as in gastroschisis) and the cord inserts upon the omphalocele sac (curved arrow). The fetus also had choroid plexus cysts (not shown). (B-bladder).

Key Facts
- Synonym: Edwards syndrome, T18
- Definition: Autosomal trisomy of chromosome 18
- Classic imaging appearance: Second trimester fetus with **multiple anomalies** involving multiple organ systems
- **Choroid plexus cyst (CPC)**: Ultrasound marker for T18
  - o 1/3 T18 fetuses have CPC (+ other anomalies)
  - o 2% of normal fetuses have isolated CPC (- other anomalies)
  - o CPC resolve in 3rd trimester
- Dismal prognosis: 90% fatal
- Second most common autosomal trisomy
- Increased risk for T18 in advanced maternal age (> 35 yo)
- Maternal serum screen for T18

Imaging Findings
General Features
- Best imaging clue: **Multiple anomalies including T18 minor markers** for example
  - o CPC + bowel-containing omphalocele + early symmetric intrauterine growth restriction (IUGR)
  - o Strawberry shaped calvarium + rockerbottom feet
  - o Spina bifida + cystic hygroma + cardiac anomaly
Ultrasound Findings
- 80% have detectable 2nd trimester anomalies
  - o Usually multiple anomalies are seen
- Major anomalies associated with T18
  - o **Cardiac defects** (90%): 38% seen prenatally, 90% at autopsy
    - ▪ Ventricular septal defect (VSD), atrial septal defect (ASD), dextrocardia
  - o **IUGR** (51%): Early IUGR in 28% (14-24 weeks)

Trisomy 18

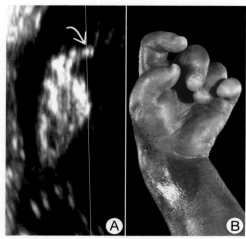

Trisomy 18. (A) Ultrasound image of the classic appearance of clenched hand with overlapping index finger (curved arrow) in a fetus with trisomy 18. (B) Gross pathology correlation.

- o Cystic hygroma (20%)
- o GI anomalies
  - **Bowel-containing omphalocele** (21%): Usually small
  - Diaphragmatic hernia
- o Meningomyelocele/spina bifida: (17%)
- o Renal (15%): Hydronephrosis most common
- Minor anomalies associated with T18
  - o Intracranial findings
    - CPC (33%)
    - Strawberry shaped calvarium: Lateral calvarial bulge
    - Large cisterna magna
    - Ventriculomegaly
    - Agenesis of the corpus callosum
  - o Two vessel umbilical cord: Single umbilical artery
  - o Musculoskeletal findings
    - **Clenched hands** with overlapping index finger
    - Clubfeet or **rockerbottom feet**
    - Short radial ray
  - o Facial anomalies
    - Micrognathia
    - Low set ears
    - Hypertelorism

Imaging Recommendations
- Careful fetal survey if any minor or major anomalies seen
- Formal fetal echocardiography
- **When CPC seen, look carefully at fetal hands and fetal heart**

Differential Diagnosis
Isolated Fetal Anomaly
- Anomaly seen is not associated with T18

293

Trisomy 18

- Isolated CPC
  - Seen in 2% of all fetuses
  - Risk for T18 **< 1:400**
  - Amniocentesis usually not done in low risk patients

Pena Shokeir Syndrome (Pseudo-Trisomy 18)
- Neurogenic arthrogryposis
- IUGR, clenched hands, multiple joint contractures
- Autosomal recessive inheritance
- 92% die within first month of life

Smith-Lemli-Opitz Syndrome
- Clenched hands, IUGR, microcephaly, abnormal genitalia
- Autosomal recessive inheritance
- Type II is lethal

Triploidy
- Multiple anomalies: Severe early IUGR, abnormal placenta
- Complete extra set of chromosomes
- Fatal

Trisomy 9
- Multiple anomalies: IUGR, microcephaly, cleft lip and palate
- Autosomal trisomic syndrome
- Usually fatal, survivors with severe mental and motor retardation

Pathology
General
- Genetics
  - Autosomal trisomic syndrome
- Epidemiology
  - Second most common autosomal trisomy: Trisomy 21 is first
  - Incidence: 1:3,000 births
  - Increased incidence in **advanced maternal age**

Clinical Issues
Presentation
- Fetus with anomalies: particularly CPC
  - Genetic counseling important when anomalies seen
- **Abnormal maternal serum triple screen result**
  - Low alpha-fetoprotein (AFP), estriol, human chorionic gondaotropin (hCG)
- Amniocentesis not done for isolated CPC in low-risk women
  - Maternal age and triple screen test are best predictors of risk

Treatment
- Majority terminate pregnancy once diagnosis is made

Prognosis
- Fetuses often die in utero
- 90% live-borns die in first year of life
- Survivors are severely retarded and handicapped

Selected References
1. Gupta JK et al: Clinical significance of fetal choroids plexus cysts. Lancet 346:724-9, 1995
2. Nyberg et al: Prenatal sonographic findings in trisomy 18: Review of 47 cases. J Ultrasound Med 2:103-13, 1993
3. Benacerraf B et al: Sonographic detection of fetuses with trisomies 13 and 18: Accuracy and limitations. Am J Obstet Gynecol 158:404-9, 1988

Trisomy 13

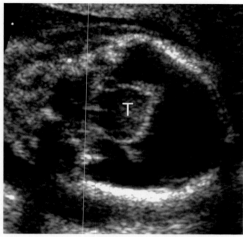

Holoprosencephaly in a fetus with trisomy 13. Oblique coronal image of the fetal head shows fused thalami (T) surround by a single horseshoe-shaped ventricle. Also note, the falx is absent. Facial images showed a proboscis and severe hypotelorism.

Key Facts
- Synonym: Patau Syndrome
- Definition: Autosomal trisomy of chromosome 13
- Classic imaging appearance: Fetus with **multiple anomalies** involving multiple organ systems; most markedly central nervous system and facial anomalies
- **Holoprosencephaly** is classic anomaly of trisomy 13 (T13)
- Dismal prognosis: 95% fatal
- Third most common autosomal trisomy

Imaging Findings
General Features
- Best imaging clue: **Midline anomalies of brain and face** as well as echogenic kidneys, polydactyly, and cardiac defects
Ultrasound Findings
- > 90% have detectable second trimester anomalies
- Central nervous system and cranial anomalies (70%)
  - Holoprosencephaly (40%): Lobar, semilobar and alobar
    - Failure of division of cerebral hemispheres and ventricles
    - Fused thalami
    - Absent cavum septi pellucidi, variable presence of falx
    - Most with an associated facial anomaly
  - Agenesis of corpus callosum
  - Cerebellar anomalies
    - Dandy-Walker malformation/variant
    - Cerebellar hypoplasia with mega cisterna magna
  - Ventriculomegaly
  - Microcephaly
- Facial Anomalies (50%)
  - Present in 80% of fetuses with CNS anomalies

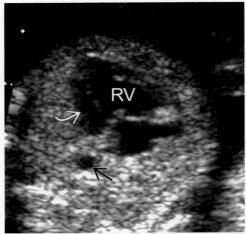

Hypoplastic left heart in the same fetus with trisomy 13. The left ventricle (curved arrow) is markedly hypoplastic when compared to the normal-sized right ventricle (RV). This fetus also had IUGR. (Black arrow – descending aorta).

- o **Midline or bilateral cleft lip +/- cleft palate**
  - ▪ Premaxillary protrusion seen on profile views
- o **Cyclopia** or hypotelorism (36%)
- o **Proboscis**: Tube-like nose, often superior to orbits, profile view best
- Extremity anomalies (50%)
  - o Post axial **polydactyly** (75%)
  - o Club/rockerbottom feet
  - o Clenched hand/overlapping digits
- Intrauterine growth restriction (**IUGR**) in 50%
  - o **IUGR + polyhydramnios should raise suspicion for T13 and T18**
- Renal anomalies (50%)
  - o **Echogenic kidneys**: Cystic dysplasia
  - o Hydronephrosis
- Cardiac defects (50%)
  - o Hypoplastic left heart
  - o Ventricular septal defect
- Gastrointestinal anomalies
  - o Omphalocele: Usually contains bowel +/- liver
  - o Echogenic bowel
- Minor markers for T13: almost never isolated
  - o Intracardiac echogenic focus (30%)
  - o Single umbilical artery (25%)
  - o Increased nuchal thickening/ translucency (20%)
  - o Echogenic bowel (5%)

Other Modality Findings
- Fetal MR can help diagnose subtle CNS defects
  - o Agenesis of corpus callosum, absence of cavum septi pellucidi

Imaging Recommendations
- Suspect brain anomaly when midline facial anomalies are seen
  - o "The face predicts the brain"

- Consider fetal MR when CNS findings are minimal

Differential Diagnosis
Meckel-Gruber Syndrome
- Encephalocele, polydactyly, enlarged echogenic kidneys
- Holoprosencephaly and Dandy-Walker sometimes seen
- Autosomal recessive with 25% recurrence risk
Holoprosencephaly Without T13
- Less severe cases are compatible with life

Pathology
General
- Genetics
  o Autosomal trisomic syndrome
- Epidemiology
  o 1:6,000 births
  o Less common than trisomy 21 and trisomy 18
  o Associated with advanced maternal age

Clinical Issues
Presentation
- Fetus with multiple anomalies: Particularly holoprosencephaly
  o Genetic counseling and amniocentesis
- Maternal serum screen may show low alpha-fetoprotein (AFP)
Treatment
- Majority terminate pregnancy once diagnosis is made
Prognosis
- Some die in utero but most survive to birth
- 75% die in first 6 months of life
- Less than 5% survive beyond three years of life

Selected References
1. Tongsong T et al: Sonographic features of trisomy 13 at midpregnancy. Int J Gynecol Obstet 76:143-8, 2001
2. Lehman CD et al: Trisomy 13 syndrome: Prenatal US findings in a review of 33 cases. Radiology 194:217-22, 1995
3. Nicolaidies KH et al: Ultrasonographically detectable markers of fetal chromosomal abnormalities. Lancet 340:704-7, 1992

Turner Syndrome

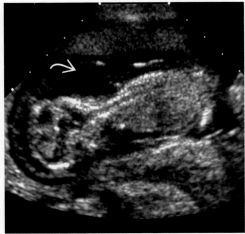

Turner syndrome. 14 week fetus with a cystic hygroma (arrow) and hydrops. Note marked skin edema surrounding fetus. There was in utero demise on an ultrasound 2 weeks later. Chromosomal analysis confirmed 45X karyotype.

Key Facts
- Synonyms: Monosomy X, 45X
- Definition: Genetic disorder due to **absence of one sex chromosome**
- Classic imaging appearance: Female fetus with nuchal cystic hygroma (CH) often hydrops +/- other structural anomalies
- Most common chromosome abnormality when CH seen
- Majority of fetuses with Turner syndrome (TS) **die in utero**
- Not associated with advanced maternal age
- **Increased nuchal translucency** may be seen in first trimester
- Abnormalities of lymphatic drainage cause most anomalies seen

Imaging Findings
General Features
- Best imaging clue: 1st or 2nd trimester **female fetus with septated cystic hygroma and hydrops +/- cardiac anomaly**
Ultrasound Findings
- Nuchal cystic hygroma in second trimester
  - o Characteristic anomaly of TS
  - o Fluid collection involving posterior and lateral neck
  - o Usually large and obvious
    - ▪ May be confused with pockets of amniotic fluid
  - o Contains several thin septations
- Increased nuchal translucency in first trimester
  - o Neck skin lucency > 3 mm considered abnormal
  - o If septations, then more suspicious for TS than trisomy 21
  - o May see associated hydrops in first trimester
- **Non-immune hydrops**
  - o Excess fetal fluid accumulates in skin and body cavities
  - o Skin edema: Lymphangiectasia

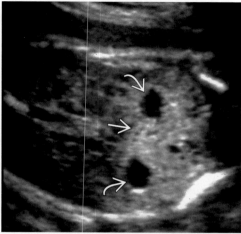

Turner syndrome. Coronal image through the abdomen of a fetus with Turner syndrome. There is a horseshoe kidney with an isthmus of tissue crossing the midline (arrow). There is mild bilateral pelviectasis (curved arrows).

- o Bilateral pleural effusions
- o Ascites
- o Pericardial effusion: Especially if cardiac anomaly present
- Cardiovascular anomalies (25%)
  - o **Coarctation of aorta**: Most common
    - May be difficult diagnosis in utero
    - Secondary signs include small left ventricle
- Genitourinary anomalies
  - o **Horseshoe kidney**
    - Kidneys are fused inferiorly
    - Isthmus of renal tissue lies anterior to aorta
    - Seen best on transverse and coronal views
    - May be difficult diagnosis in utero
  - o Ambiguous genitalia (rare)
  - o Ovarian dysgenesis: Not diagnosed in utero
- Short limbs
  - o Mild short femur and humerus length

Imaging Recommendations
- May need high gain settings to see septations within CH
- Note gender of fetus when CH is seen
- Measure fluid carefully, large CH can mimic amniotic fluid
- Consider **formal fetal echocardiography** to look for aortic coarctation

Differential Diagnosis

Cystic Hygroma Without Turner Syndrome
- Also seen with trisomy 21, trisomy 18 and normal chromosomes
- 2/3 of all CH associated with chromosome abnormality

Noonan Syndrome
- Phenotypical features similar to Turner syndrome
- Karyotype is normal

Turner Syndrome

- Occurs in males and females
- Autosomal dominant condition in some patients

Pathology
General
- Genetics
  - Karyotype is **45X**
  - Paternal sex chromosome usually absent
  - Mosaic 45X seen in 15% of cases
  - Partial abnormality of one sex chromosome can lead to TS phenotype
- Etiology-Pathogenesis
  - Failure/delayed connection between internal jugular veins and lymph sacs
  - Hydrops from fluid overload secondary to lymphatic failure
- Epidemiology
  - 25% all spontaneous abortions from chromosome abnormality are 45X
  - 9% of all 1st trimester abortions are 45X
  - Live birth rate is 1:3,000 female births
  - **Not** associated with advanced maternal age

Clinical Issues
Presentation
- Fetal anomalies: Particularly CH
- Abnormal maternal biochemical screen
  - 53% detection rate
  - Very low estriol
  - Low alpha-fetoprotein
  - Human chorionic gonadotropin (hCG)
    - Elevated if hydrops present
    - Low without hydrops
  - Inhibin
    - Elevated if hydrops present
    - Low without hydrops
Natural History
- Majority of TS spontaneously abort or die in 2nd trimester
Prognosis
- Dismal if hydrops develops
- Prognosis depends on associated anomalies
- Mosaic TS (15%) with better prognosis
- Survivors
  - Webbed neck, short stature, infertile, horseshoe kidney, narrow maxilla, small mandible, cubitus valgus
  - Normal verbal IQ
  - Delayed motor skills

Selected References
1. Gravholr CH et al: Prenatal and postnatal prevalence of Turner's syndrome: A registry study. BMJ 312:16-21, 1996
2. Saller DN et al: Multiple-marker screening in pregnancies with hydrops and non-hydropic Turner syndrome. Am J Obstet Gynecol 167:1021-4, 1992
3. Phillips HE et al: Intrauterine fetal cystic hygroma: Sonographic detection. AJR 136:799-802, 1981

Triploidy

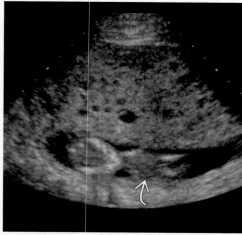

Triploidy. Longitudinal scan of the uterus of a 14 week pregnancy shows a markedly enlarged, heterogeneous, cystic-appearing placenta. There is oligohydramnios and a small fetus crowded posteriorly (curved arrow).

Key Facts
- Synonym: Partial mole
- Definition: 69 chromosomes (one entire extra haploid set)
  - Extra set usually paternal
- Classic imaging appearance: Fetus with **severe intrauterine growth restriction (IUGR), abnormal placenta, and multiple anomalies**
- Common chromosomal anomaly in 1st trimester miscarriages
- Most miscarry before 20 weeks
- **Not** related to maternal age

Imaging Findings
General Features
- Best imaging clue: **Early asymmetric IUGR**
Ultrasound Findings
- Increased nuchal translucency in 1st trimester
- Severe IUGR
  - Early onset
    - Can be diagnosed by 11 weeks
  - Asymmetric distribution
    - Abdomen most profoundly affected
- **Placenta** often abnormal (variable appearance)
  - **Large, hydropic, heterogeneous**
    - Extra haploid chromosome set **paternal**
  - **Small, calcified**
    - Extra haploid chromosome set **maternal**
- **CNS**
  - **Ventriculomegaly**
  - Dandy-Walker malformation
  - Agenesis of corpus callosum
  - Holoprosencephaly

Triploidy

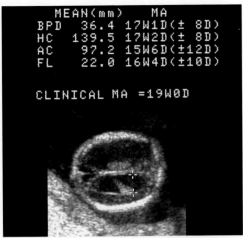

```
       MEAN(mm)      MA
BPD    36.4   17W1D(±  8D)
HC    139.5   17W2D(±  8D)
AC     97.2   15W6D(±12D)
FL     22.0   16W4D(±10D)


CLINICAL MA =19W0D
```

Triploidy. Fetal biometry shows early asymmetric IUGR with the abdomen most severely affected. Ventriculomegaly (cursors) as well as other anomalies were identified. Amniocentesis confirmed 69XXX karyotype.

- Other associated anomalies
  - Omphalocele
    - Small bowel containing
  - Cystic hygroma
  - Hydronephrosis and renal dysplasia
  - **Cardiac defects**
  - Clubbed feet
  - **Syndactyly 3rd and 4th digit**
  - Micrognathia
- Oligohydramnios frequent
- Ovarian theca lutein cysts sometimes seen

Imaging Recommendations
- Abnormal-appearing placenta should raise high suspicion
- Perform endovaginal for fetal anatomy
- Short follow-up interval in 1st trimester (7-10 days)
  - IUGR and anomalies seen early

Differential Diagnosis

Hydatidiform Mole With Coexistent Fetus
- Living fetus will have a separate normal appearing placenta
- Fetus should have normal anatomy and growth

Demise With Hydropic Degeneration Of Placenta
- Represents hydropic change without trophoblastic proliferation
- Can look identical and pathologist must make diagnosis
- Low human chorionic gonadotropin (hCG) levels

Placental Pseudomoles
- Mesenchymal dysplasia of placenta results in villus hydrops
- Often seen with pre-eclampsia and normal fetus
- May be seen with placentomegaly and Beckwith-Wiedeman syndrome

Triploidy

Trisomies 18,13
- Many fetal findings overlap
- Placenta is usually normal
- IUGR does not manifest as early

Neu-Laxova Syndrome
- Early IUGR
- Ichthyosis
- Severe microcephaly

Pathology
General
- Genetics
  - Sporadic
- Etiology-Pathogenesis
  - Diandry: Extra chromosome set paternal (70-90%)
    - Fertilization with 2 sperm most common (dispermy)
    - Fertilization with diploid sperm
  - Digyny: Extra chromosome set maternal
    - Diploid egg
- Epidemiology
  - 1-2% of conceptions
  - 30% of 1st trimester abortuses

Clinical Issues
Presentation
- Anomalies and IUGR seen in 1st trimester
- Laboratory abnormalities vary according to source of extra chromosomes
  - Paternal: Increased hCG, alpha-fetoprotein (AFP)
  - Maternal: Low hCG, AFP, estriol

Natural History
- Most spontaneously abort before 20 weeks

Treatment
- Chorionic villus sampling or amniocentesis for karyotype
- Termination offered

Prognosis
- Lethal

Selected References
1. Genest DR Partial hydatidiform mole: Clinicopathological features, differential diagnosis, ploidy and molecular studies, and gold standards for diagnosis. Int J Gynecol Pathol 20:315-22, 2001
2. Jauniaux E et al: Partial mole and triploidy: Screening patients with first-trimester spontaneous abortion. Obstet Gynecol 88:616-9, 1996
3. Jauniaux E et al: Prenatal diagnosis of triploidy during the second trimester of pregnancy. Obstet Gynecol 88:983-9, 1996

PocketRadiologist®
Obstetrics
Top 100 Diagnoses

SYNDROMES

Meckel-Gruber Syndrome

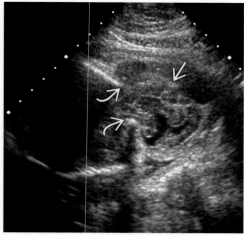

Meckel-Gruber syndrome. Sonographic image of the fetal cranium shows an encephalocele with a large skull defect (curved arrows) and herniation of brain tissue (arrow).

Key Facts
- Synonym: Dysencephalia splanchnocystica
- Definition: **Autosomal recessive** disorder characterized by
  - Encephalocele 60-80%
  - Renal cystic dysplasia 100%
  - Postaxial polydactyly 55-75%
- Classic imaging appearance: Fetus with enlarged echogenic kidneys, encephalocele, and polydactyly
- Wide phenotypic variation
- Diagnosis can confidently be made between 11-14 weeks
- **Lethal** malformation

Imaging Findings
General Features
- Best imaging clue: **At least 2 of 3** classics features in fetus with normal karyotype
Ultrasound Findings
- CNS
  - **Encephalocele**
    - Variable size
    - Occipital
  - Microcephaly common
  - Dandy-Walker malformation
  - Agenesis of corpus callosum
  - Ventriculomegaly
- Kidneys
  - **Renal cystic dysplasia most consistent finding**
  - Large size
  - Vary from diffusely echogenic (microscopic cysts) to macroscopic cysts
  - Bladder may be small or absent

Meckel-Gruber Syndrome

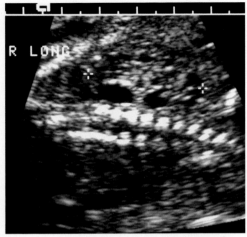

Meckel-Gruber syndrome. Image of the right kidney in the same fetus shows cystic dysplasia (cursors). It is enlarged and echogenic with several discrete macroscopic cysts (the left kidney had a similar appearance). Visualization was difficult secondary to associated oligohydramnios.

- o **2nd trimester oligohydramnios**
- Extremities
  - o **Postaxial polydactyly**
    - ▪ May be difficult to see if oligohydramnios
    - ▪ Extra digit may be small or angulated
  - o Clubbed feet common
  - o Short limbs
- Facial malformation
  - o Cleft lip/palate
  - o Micrognathia
  - o Microphthalmia
  - o Ear malformations
- Cardiac
  - o Septal defects
  - o Coarctation
- Other anomalies
  - o **Hepatic fibrosis**
    - ▪ Universally seen at autopsy
    - ▪ Difficult to appreciate in utero
    - ▪ Look for hepatomegaly and poor intrahepatic flow
  - o Cryptorchidism
  - o Hypoplastic genitalia

Imaging Recommendations
- Look for associated findings
- MRI helpful if oligohydramnios limits visualization

Differential Diagnosis
Trisomy 13
- Kidneys usually small

Meckel-Gruber Syndrome

- Holoprosencephaly
- Encephalocele reported but less common

Pathology
General
- Genetics
  - Autosomal recessive
  - Linked to chromosomes 17q and 11q
- Etiology-Pathogenesis: Postulated
  - Failure of mesodermal induction
- Epidemiology
  - 0.1-0.7 in 10,000 births
  - Finnish population 1:9,000
  - 5% of neural tube defects

Clinical Issues
Presentation
- May have prior history
- Elevated maternal serum alpha-fetoprotein
- Small-for-dates secondary to oligohydramnios
Natural History
- Oligohydramnios leads to pulmonary hypoplasia
- Most stillborn or die within a few hours
Treatment
- Karyotype to exclude trisomy 13
- Termination offered
- External examination and autopsy by experienced pathologist/geneticist to confirm diagnosis
- Genetic counseling for future pregnancies
Prognosis
- Lethal
- **25% recurrence risk**

Selected References
1. Sepulveda W et al: Diagnosis of the Meckel-Gruber syndrome at eleven to fourteen weeks gestation. Am J Obstet Gynecol 176:316-9, 1997
2. Nyberg DA et al: Meckel-Gruber syndrome. Importance of prenatal diagnosis. J Ultrasound Med 9:691-6, 1990
3. Salonen R The Meckel syndrome: Clinicopathological findings in 67 patients. Am J Med Genet 18:671-89, 1984

VACTERL Association

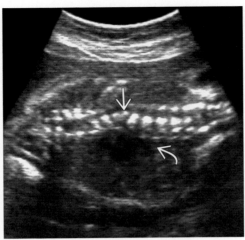

VACTERL association. Coronal sonogram of the spine shows scoliosis secondary to fused vertebrae (arrow). There is also a multicystic dysplastic kidney (curved arrow). This was bilateral resulting in anhydramnios making visualization difficult. At autopsy there was also esophageal atresia and a ventricular septal defect.

Key Facts
- Synonym: VATER, VACTER syndrome
- Definition: Non-random association of anomalies including
  - Vertebral anomalies
  - Anal atresia
  - Cardiac malformations
  - Tracheo-Esophgeal fistula
  - Renal anomalies
  - Limb malformation
  - Debated whether 2 or 3 findings are needed for diagnosis
- Classic imaging appearance: Multiple anomalies involving multiple organ systems
- **CNS malformations not** a feature of this association
  - VACTERL + hydrocephalus (VACTERL-H) considered separate entity with worse prognosis

Imaging Findings
General Features
- Best imaging clue: **Renal and vertebral** anomalies most easily identified
Ultrasound Findings
- Vertebral anomalies
  - Hemivertebrae
    - Kyphosis
    - Scoliosis
    - Best demonstrated in coronal plane
  - Butterfly vertebrae
  - Fusion of vertebral bodies or posterior elements (block vertebrae)
  - Caudal regression
- Anal atresia
  - Normal anus is echogenic ring

VACTERL Association

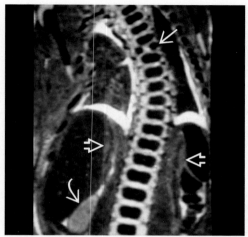

VACTERL association. Postmortem T2WI coronal image shows a butterfly vertebra and scoliosis (arrow). There was renal agenesis giving the adrenal glands an abnormal elongated appearance (open arrows). There was also anal atresia with partial visualization of a dilated bowel loop in the renal fossa (curved arrow).

- o Absent in atresia
- o Colon can occasionally be dilated
- o May not be recognized prenatally
- Cardiac malformations
- Tracheoesophageal fistula
  - o Stomach absent or small
  - o Most common anomaly in VACTERL association
    - ▪ Often difficult to diagnose
- Renal anomalies
  - o Multicystic dysplastic kidney
  - o Hydronephrosis
  - o Agenesis
- Limb malformation
  - o **Radial ray malformation common**
  - o Abnormal hands
    - ▪ Polydactyly
    - ▪ Syndactyly
- Fluid variable
  - o Most often **polyhydramnios** secondary to esophageal atresia
  - o Oligohydramnios with bilateral renal anomalies
- Other associated malformations
  - o Intrauterine growth restriction (IUGR)
  - o Single umbilical artery
  - o Cleft lip/palate
  - o Rib anomalies

Imaging Recommendations
- If one defect in association identified targeted search for other anomalies
- Dedicated fetal echo

VACTERL Association

Differential Diagnosis
Trisomy 18,13
- **CNS malformations** common
- Many overlapping features VACTERL association
- All fetuses should be karyotyped

Syndromes With Overlapping Findings
- Holt-Oram (heart-hand syndrome)
- Thrombocytopenia absent radius (TAR)
- Roberts syndrome (pseudothalidomide)
- Jarcho-Levin syndrome (vertebral, rib anomalies)

Pathology
General
- Genetics
  - Sporadic
  - Not associated with chromosomal abnormality but shares many common features
  - **VACTERL-H**
    - Separate entity
    - **X-linked and autosomal recessive**
    - **Poor prognosis**
    - **Severe retardation**
- Etiology-Pathogenesis
  - Abnormal mesodermal development (mechanism unknown)
  - Risk factors: Maternal diabetes
- Epidemiology
  - 1:10,000 in prenatal series

Clinical Issues
Presentation
- Multiple malformations on routine scan

Treatment
- **Karyotype to rule out trisomy**
- Termination offered
  - Autopsy encouraged to establish diagnosis
- Delivery at tertiary care facility if pregnancy continued

Prognosis
- Variable based on type and number of anomalies
  - 28% neonatal mortality
- Intelligence usually normal unless VACTERL-H

Selected References
1. Miller OF et al: Prenatal diagnosis of VACTERL association. J Urol 166:2389-91, 2001
2. Tongsong T et al: Prenatal sonographic diagnosis of VATER association. J Clin Ultrasound 27:378-84, 1999
3. Froster UG et al: VACTERL with hydrocephalus and branchial arch defects: Prenatal, clinical, and autopsy findings in two brothers. Am J Med Genet 62:169-72, 1996

PocketRadiologist®
Obstetrics
Top 100 Diagnoses

MISCELLANEOUS

Polyhydramnios

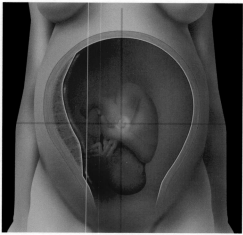

Polyhydramnios. Excessive fluid surrounds the fetus and distends the uterus. The uterus can be divided into quadrants and the sum of the largest pockets of fluid in each quadrant determines the amniotic fluid index.

Key Facts
- Synonym: Hydramnios
- Definition: Excessive amniotic fluid
- Classic imaging appearance: Fetus is surrounded by an abundance of amniotic fluid (AF)
- Polyhydramnios is common (1-4% of all pregnancies)
- **2/3 of cases are idiopathic** and mild (diagnosis of exclusion)
- 1/3 of cases are associated with **fetal anomaly or maternal diabetes**
- Likelihood of fetal anomaly increases with severity of polyhydramnios
- May be an early sign of hydrops or twin-twin transfusion
- Can cause preterm labor when severe

Imaging Findings
General Features
- Best imaging clue
  - 2nd trimester: AF to baby ratio is greater than 1:1
  - 3rd trimester: Significantly increased AF seen between uterine wall and fetus

Ultrasound Findings
- Experienced sonographers can subjectively detect increased AF accurately
- **Semiquantitative measurements** of AF confirms diagnosis
- Maximum vertical pocket (MVP) measurement
  - Largest pocket of AF free of fetal parts and umbilical cord found
  - Measurement is in vertical plane (anterior-posterior measurement)
  - Use **color Doppler** to avoid measuring umbilical cord
  - Polyhydramnios if > 8 cm (normal is 2-8 cm)
- **Amniotic fluid index (AFI)** measurement
  - Uterus divided into 4 equal quadrants
  - Sum of MVP in each quadrant = AFI
  - **Polyhydramnios if AFI > 20 cm**

Polyhydramnios

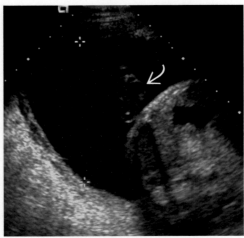

Polyhydramnios. A maximum vertical pocket of fluid is measured (calipers). Notice that the umbilical cord (curved arrow) is not included in the measurement. This is a case of mild idiopathic polyhydramnios.

- Two diameter pocket (TDP) measurement
  - Vertical and horizontal measurements of largest pocket are multiplied
  - Polyhydramnios if TDP > 50 cm² (normal is 15-50 cm²)
- 1/3 of cases have an associated finding
  - **Fetal macrosomia** (with or without diabetes mellitus)
  - Hydrops from any cause
  - **Fetal gastrointestinal (GI) anomalies**
    - Atresias: Esophageal, duodenal, jejunal/ileal
    - Abdominal wall defects: Gastroschisis, omphalocele
    - Diaphragmatic hernia
  - **Fetal central nervous system (CNS) anomalies**
    - Impaired swallowing from any CNS cause
    - Neural tube defects: anencephaly, encephalocele, spina bifida
    - Hydrocephalus, microcephaly, Dandy-Walker malformation
  - Fetal cardiovascular system anomalies
    - Arrhythmia, congenital anomaly, cardiac tumors
  - Fetal respiratory system anomaly
    - Chest mass, tracheal atresia, pleural effusion
  - Fetal musculoskeletal anomaly: Likely related to fetal skin AF pathways
    - Skeletal dysplasia
    - Any impairment of fetal movement
  - Twin-twin transfusion

Imaging Recommendations
- Look carefully for fetal anomalies and fetal growth
- Look for a stuck twin as in twin-twin transfusion
- Idiopathic polyhydramnios is a diagnosis of exclusion

Differential Diagnosis
Normal AF
- AF may transiently seem increased but normalize with follow-up

Polyhydramnios

Pathology
<u>General</u>
- Etiology-Pathogenesis
  - AF volume regulation reflects balance between production and removal
  - Major AF production
    - **Fetal kidneys: 800-1200 cc/day** near term,
    - Fetal lungs: 170 cc/day near term
  - Major AF removal
    - Fetal swallowing/intestines: 500-1000 cc/day near term
    - Fetal lungs: 170 cc/day near term
  - Other major AF transfer pathways
    - Placenta, membranes, fetal skin, umbilical cord
  - Abnormalities of fetal anatomy, fetal movement, fetal size or other transfer pathways can affect AF balance

Clinical Issues
<u>Presentation</u>
- Incidentally noted during routine obstetrical examination: Idiopathic
  - Common
  - Follow-up exam performed but genetic amniocentesis not necessary
- Maternal diabetes mellitus

<u>Natural History</u>
- Severe polyhydramnios associated with **preterm labor**, premature rupture of membranes, placental abruption
- May stay mild and chronic or become acutely increased

<u>Treatment</u>
- Karyotype indicated for suspicious fetal anomalies or in cases of polyhdyramnios with intrauterine growth restriction
- **Therapeutic amniocentesis**
- Indomethacin
  - Rapid placental passage
  - Decreases both fetal urinary tract and lung fluid output
  - Reduction of fluid within 1 week
  - Effective in > 90%
  - Side effect: Potential constriction of ductus arteriosus

<u>Prognosis</u>
- Depends on cause for polyhydramnios
- Idiopathic has excellent prognosis

Selected References
1. Mcgann EF et al: The amniotic fluid index, single deepest pocket, and two diameter pocket in normal human pregnancy. Am J Obstet Gynecol 182:1581-8, 2000
2. Moise KJ: Polyhydramnios. Clin Obstet Gynecol 40: 266-79, 1997
3. Many A, et al: The association between polyhydramnios and preterm delivery. Obstet Gynecol 86:389-91, 1995

Oligohydramnios

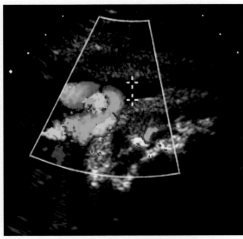

Oligohydramnios. A small pocket of fluid is measured (calipers) in this pregnancy complicated by premature rupture of membranes. This was the largest pocket of fluid seen. Note how color Doppler is used in order to avoid measuring the umbilical cord.

Key Facts
- Synonym: Anhydramnios (no detectable fluid)
- Definition: Deficiency of amniotic fluid
- Classic imaging appearance: **Fetal crowding** and lack of normal pockets of amniotic fluid (AF)
- Unlike polyhydramnios, **idiopathic oligohydramnios is rare** (<1%)
- Associated with **fetal urinary tract anomalies**
- Seen commonly with intrauterine growth restriction (**IUGR**)
- Most important finding in abnormal biophysical profile score testing
- May be an early indicator of fetal hypoxia
- Severe and chronic oligohydramnios associated with poor prognosis predominately due to pulmonary hypoplasia
- Transient and late oligohydramnios has good outcome

Imaging Findings
General Features
- Best imaging clue: Fetus seems confined and anatomy is difficult to see when severe
Ultrasound Findings
- Experienced sonographers can subjectively detect decreased AF
- **Semiquantitative measurements of AF** confirms diagnosis
- Maximum vertical pocket (MVP) measurement
  - Largest pocket of AF free of fetal parts and umbilical cord found
  - Measurement is in vertical plane (anterior-posterior measurement)
  - Use color Doppler to avoid measuring umbilical cord
  - Oligohydramnios if < 2 cm (normal is 2-8 cm)
- **Amniotic fluid index** (AFI) measurement
  - Uterus divided into 4 equal quadrants
  - Sum of MVP in each quadrant = AFI
  - **Oligohydramnios if AFI < 5 cm**

Oligohydramnios

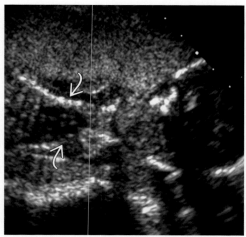

Oligohydramnios. Note lack of fluid and compressive effect of the uterus upon the fetal chest (arrows).

- Two diameter pocket (TDP) measurement
  - Vertical and horizontal measurements of largest pocket are multiplied
  - Oligohydramnios if TDP < 15 cm² (normal is 15-50 cm²)
- Fluid measurement for biophysical profile score
  - Score of 2 = pocket of fluid > 2 cm in two perpendicular planes
  - **Score of 0 = no 2 cm x 2 cm pocket of fluid**
- Anomalies associated with oligohydramnios (20% of all cases)
  - Urinary tract anomalies most common (60%)
    - **Renal agenesis**, bladder outlet obstruction, bilateral multicystic renal dysplasia, autosomal recessive polycystic kidney disease
    - Color Doppler of renal arteries helps rules out renal agenesis
    - **Amniotic fluid may be present early in pregnancy**
  - Multiple anomalies present in 10%
  - Confined fetus at risk for **limb and facial deformities**
    - Clubfoot, Potter facies
- IUGR (20-40% of all cases)
  - Estimated fetal weight is < 10th percentile
  - Cord Doppler waveform may show increased resistance
- **Post-term pregnancy**
  - Gestational age > 42 weeks
- **Premature rupture of membranes** (PROM)
  - Poor prognosis when early (< 25 weeks) and prolonged (> 14 days)

Imaging Recommendations
- Look carefully for fetal anomalies and IUGR
- May need transvaginal ultrasound (TVUS)
  - TVUS contraindicated with premature ruptured membranes (PROM)
- Fetal MRI preferable to amnioinfusion for better anatomic visualization
- **Frequent follow up (1-2 x/wk) in borderline cases**

Oligohydramnios

Differential Diagnosis
Normal AF
- Oligohydramnios may be mild and transient
- May be related to maternal hydration status and improve

Pathology
General
- Etiology-Pathogenesis
  - AF volume regulation reflects balance between production and removal
  - Major AF production
    - **Fetal kidneys: 800-1200 cc/day** near term,
    - Fetal lungs: 170 cc/day near term
  - Major AF removal
    - Fetal swallowing/intestines: 500-1000 cc/day near term
    - Fetal lungs: 170 cc/day near term
  - Other major AF transfer pathways
    - Placenta, membranes, fetal skin, umbilical cord
  - Abnormalities of fetal anatomy, movement, size or other transfer pathways can affect AF balance

Clinical Issues
Presentation
- Incidentally noted during routine obstetrical examination
- Associated with fetal genitourinary anomaly
- PROM or post-date pregnancy
- Associated with twin-twin transfusion

Treatment
- Maternal hydration
  - Not helpful if due to fetal anomaly or PROM
- Bed rest if due to poor placental function
- Amnioinfusion during active labor
  - Decreases risk of cord compression

Prognosis
- Depends on cause of oligohydramnios and time of presentation
  - **Less than 25 weeks associated with 10% survival rate**
  - Isolated 3rd trimester oligohydramnios with good outcome
- Dismal if from bilateral renal anomaly
- Second trimester oligohydramnios associated with pulmonary hypoplasia
- Worse prognosis if duration of oligohydramnios > 14 days

Selected References
1. Mcgann EF et al: The amniotic fluid index, single deepest pocket, and two diameter pocket in normal human pregnancy. Am J Obstet Gynecol 182:1581-8, 2000
2. Shipp TD et al: Outcome of singleton pregnancies with severe oligohydramnios in the second and third trimester. Ultrasound Obstet Gynecol 7:108-13, 1996
3. Shenker L et al: Significance of oligohydramnios complicating pregnancy. Am J Obstet Gynecol 164:1597-1600, 1991

Hydrops

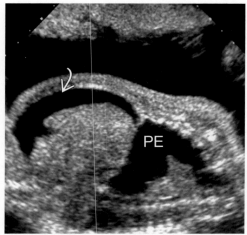

Hydrops. Sagittal view of the fetal body shows pleural effusion (PE) and ascites (arrow) in this fetus with nonimmune hydrops. Note the presence of polyhydramnios and mild skin edema.

Key Facts
- Synonyms: Hydrops fetalis
- Definition: Excess of total body fluid
- Classic imaging appearance: Ascites and pleural effusion + anasarca + polyhydramnios + placentomegaly
- 2 major categories
  - **Immune**: Fetal anemia from maternal antibodies to fetal red blood cells (usually from **maternal Rh sensitization**)
  - **Nonimmune**: Fetal fluid imbalance due to anomalies, infection, chromosome abnormality (most common)
- Maternal blood test determines immune vs nonimmune cause
- 20% of cases are idiopathic
- **40% also have detectable structural anomaly**
- Prognosis poor if not treated
- **Ultrasound features similar for immune and non-immune causes**

Imaging Findings
General Features
- Best imaging clue: **Fluid accumulation in two body cavities or one body cavity and anasarca** (skin/subcutaneous edema)
Ultrasound Findings
- Two areas of fluid accumulation required for diagnosis
- Body cavity serous effusions
  - **Ascites**: Often earliest finding with immune hydrops
  - **Pleural effusion**: Bilateral
  - Pericardial effusion: Early finding when abnormal heart
- Skin and subcutaneous thickening
  - Scalp edema often earliest most prominent area
- **Placentomegaly** from placental edema
  - > 4 cm thickness is abnormal

Hydrops

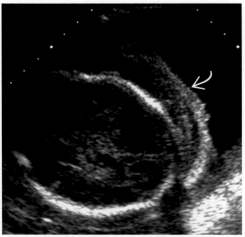

Hydrops. Transverse view of the fetal calvarium demonstrates marked scalp edema (arrow) in this fetus with anasarca.

- o Inconstant finding
- **Polyhydramnios**
  - o Can be an early isolated sign
  - o More common with immune hydrops
- Oligohydramnios
  - o Late finding with poor prognosis
- **Middle cerebral artery (MCA) Doppler**
  - o Identifies most fetuses with **anemia prior to hydrops onset**
  - o Peak systolic value obtained at 0° angle
  - o Compared with gestational age, values > 1.5 of median are abnormal
  - o Test used when anemia suspected (Rh isoimmunized patients)
- Abnormalities associated with nonimmune hydrops
  - o **Cardiac abnormalities** (30%)
    - ▪ Tachyarrhythmia: Treatable
    - ▪ Structural anomaly, poor contractility
    - ▪ Cardiac mass or mass effect upon heart
  - o Chromosome and fetal syndrome markers (16%)
    - ▪ Markers for Turner syndrome, triploidy, Noonan syndrome, myotonic dystrophy, trisomies 13, 18, 21
    - ▪ **Turner syndrome**: Cystic hygroma + hydrops
  - o Chest anomalies (6%)
    - ▪ Congenital cystic adenomatoid malformation, diaphragmatic hernia, sequestration, mass
    - ▪ Mass effect on heart obstructs venous return
  - o Infection (Parvovirus B19 most common)
    - ▪ Calcifications: Pericardial, brain, liver, peritoneal
  - o Placental chorioangioma
    - ▪ Polyhydramnios more common than hydrops

Imaging Recommendations
- Careful search for causes of nonimmune hydrops
- **M-mode of fetal heart** to rule out tachyarrhythmia

Hydrops

Differential Diagnosis
Isolated Ascites
- More likely from urinary tract obstruction or gastrointestinal perforation
- May be earliest sign of hydrops so follow-up indicated

Isolated Pericardial Effusion
- < 2 mm considered normal
- When abnormal, likely association with cardiac anomaly

Isolated Unilateral Pleural Effusion
- Chylothorax most likely

Skeletal Dysplasia With Redundant Skin
- Excess skin should not be confused with edema

Pathology
General
- Etiology-Pathogenesis
  - Immune Hydrops
    - **Fetal anemia** $\Rightarrow$ ↑cardiac output + extramedullary erythropoesis (mostly in liver)
    - Worsening anemia leads to high output heart failure + portal venous hypertension $\Rightarrow$ hydrops
    - 20-25% untreated Rh sensitized patients develop hydrops
  - Nonimmune hydrops: From variety of causes
    - Anemia from infection (like immune pathogenesis)
    - Heart failure from primary cardiac anomaly or mass effect
    - Obstruction of lymphatics (Turner syndrome)

Clinical Issues
Presentation
- Rh sensitized patient or patient exposed to Parvovirus
- Large-for-dates (polyhydramnios)

Treatment
- Immune Hydrops
  - Prior to sensitization: Rhogam
  - Once sensitized: Monitor MCA and treat anemia with **in utero transfusion (cordocentesis)**
- Nonimmune
  - Treat cause if possible
  - **Tachyarrhythmia treated pharmacologically**
  - Anemia from infection treated with in utero transfusion

Prognosis
- 75% survival for immune hydrops treated with blood transfusion
- Near 100% fatal if hydrops + fetal anomaly (excluding tachyarrhythmia)

Selected References
1. Isakaros J et al: Outcome of nonimmune hydrops fetalis diagnosed during the first half of pregnancy. Obstet Gynecol 3:321-5, 1997
2. Copel JA et al: Alloimmune disorders and pregnancy. Semin Perinatol 15:251-6, 1991
3. Mahony BS et al: Severe nonimmune hydrops fetalis: sonographic evaluation. Radiology 151:757-61, 1984

Infection

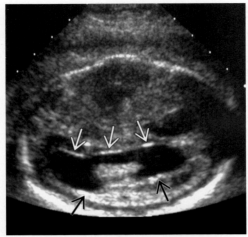

CMV infection. Axial image shows ventriculomegaly with echogenic lateral ventricular walls (arrows), which proved to be calcifications on a neonatal head CT. The head was microcephalic measuring approximately 4 weeks less than expected.

Key Facts
- Definition: Transplacental infection of fetus
- Classic imaging appearance: Multiple, variable findings which may include ventriculomegaly, calcifications (intracranial, liver), hydrops, and intrauterine growth restriction (IUGR)
- **A normal-appearing fetus does not rule out infection**
  - Maternal history, serologies, and often direct fetal testing needed for diagnosis

Imaging Findings
General Features
- Best imaging clue: **Intracranial and intrahepatic calcifications** most suspicious findings for infection
  - Calcifications are often **non-shadowing**
Ultrasound Findings (Findings Common to Many Infections)
- CNS: Brain most common affected area
  - **Ventriculomegaly, microcephaly**, cataract formation, chorioretinitis
- Hepatosplenomegaly
- IUGR and hydrops with severe disease
- Both polyhydramnios (more common with hydrops) and oligohydramnios (more common with IUGR) seen
Imaging Recommendations
- Close follow-up on all cases for complications including IUGR and hydrops

Differential Diagnosis
Cytomegalovirus
- Adult infection often asymptomatic or mononucleosis-like
- Main reservoir children under 2
- **Most common in utero infection**
  - 0.5-2% of all pregnancies

Infection

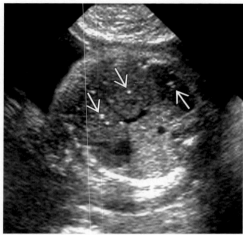

Toxoplasmosis infection. Image of the liver shows multiple, small, non-shadowing foci scattered throughout the liver (arrows).

- **Risk to fetus is greater if primary infection** while pregnant
- **30-40% fetal infection rate** from primary infection
  - **10% of these will be symptomatic**
    - 30-60% of symptomatic die within 2 years
    - 80-90% survivors have neurologic sequelae
  - 90% infected but asymptomatic in utero
    - 5-15% develop neurologic sequelae in childhood
- < 2% fetal infection rate from recurrent maternal infection
- **Calcifications common**
  - **Periventricular** and cortical
    - **Echogenic lateral ventricle** usually without shadowing
  - Liver and spleen (also hepatosplenomegaly)
- CNS: Ventriculomegaly, microcephaly
- **Echogenic bowel**

Parvovirus B19 (Fifth Disease)
- Maculopapular rash in adults
- >50% women are immune
- 20-30% transmission in infected women
- Parvovirus attacks red blood cell precursors ⇒ anemia
- **Ascites** presenting finding
- **Hydrops secondary to anemia**
  - 10-20% risk of fetal or neonatal death
  - **Treated with transfusions**
- Calcifications (intracranial and hepatic) in severe cases

Toxoplasmosis (Toxoplasma Gondii)
- Cats are definitive hosts: Oocyst shed in feces
- Human infection from contaminated soil, water, undercooked meats
- 15-40% fetal infection rate
  - Higher infection rate in 3rd trimester but not as serious
- **Intracranial calcifications**
  - **Random distribution**, echogenic non-shadowing

- **Liver calcifications** and hepatosplenomegaly

Varicella
- Primary infection chickenpox
- Latent virus in dorsal root ganglia $\Rightarrow$ shingles
- >90% women are immune
- Transmission to fetus low
- Virus affects nerve tissue $\Rightarrow$ **contractures**, limb hypoplasia
- Calcifications (liver, heart, renal), skin lesions

Herpes Simplex (Type 2)
- Most infections from vaginal delivery
- In utero infection rare
- Echogenic bowel, ventriculomegaly

Syphilis (Treponema pallidum)
- Risk of infection related to spirochete load
- Hepatosplenomegaly, dilated bowel, bowing of long bones
- Hydrops with severe cases
- 50% spontaneous abortion or perinatal death

HIV (AIDS Embryopathy)
- 20% transplacental infection
- Characteristic **craniofacial abnormalities**: Lateral bossing, hypertelorism, short nose, flat nasal bridge
- IUGR, intrauterine death in severe cases
- Amniocentesis and other **interventional procedures contraindicated**
  o Increases exposure risk to fetus

Rubella
- Rare in United States
- **Cardiac defects**, microcephaly, IUGR

Pathology
General
- Etiology-Pathogenesis
  o Early exposure increases risk to fetus
  o Infectious agents have direct cytotoxic action

Clinical Issues
Treatment
- **Thorough maternal history**
- Maternal serology
- Amniotic fluid culture
- Cordocentesis for serology and hematocrit
- Polymerase chain reaction (PCR)
  o Amplifies DNA sequence, rapid diagnosis
- Electron microscopy

Prognosis
- Varies according to infectious agent and timing, often serious
- Most long-term sequelae include hearing, visual, and neurologic abnormalities

Selected References
1. von Kaisenberg CS et al: Fetal Parvovirus B19 infection. Ultrasound Obstet Gynecol 18:280-8, 2001
2. Fowler KB et al: The outcome of congenital cytomegalovirus infection in relation to maternal antibody status. N Engl J Med 326:663-7, 1992
3. Drose JA et al: Infection in utero: US findings in 19 cases. Radiology 178:369-74, 1991

Symmetric IUGR

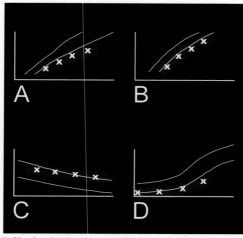

Symmetric IUGR. Graphs show biometry for fetus with all parameters small. Small fetus has grown poorly, the most ominous pattern. (A-AC, B-HC, C-HC/AC ratio, D-EFW).

Key Facts
- Synonyms: Intrauterine growth restriction (IUGR), intrauterine growth retardation, small for gestational age (SGA)
- Definition: Estimated fetal weight (EFW) < 10th percentile for gestational age (GA) with concordant head and abdominal biometry
- Classic imaging appearance: Symmetrically small fetus, often associated abnormalities
- **Accurate gestational age is key to making this diagnosis**
- Infant birth weight is single biggest factor affecting neonatal mortality
- IUGR influences morbidity and mortality at all stages of life
- Arbitrary division into symmetric/asymmetric with considerable overlap
  - Asymmetric IUGR
    - Placental problem
    - Abdominal circumference most affected
    - Onset late 2nd to 3rd trimester
    - Associated with adverse perinatal outcome
    - Outcome improved with aggressive monitoring and use of Doppler
  - Symmetric IUGR
    - Fetal problem
    - Growth restriction uniform all parameters
    - Earlier onset, even in first trimester
    - Generally gloomy prognosis
    - Outcome unlikely to improve

Imaging Findings
General Features
- Best imaging clue: Size less than expected for dates, biometric parameters equally affected
Ultrasound Findings
- Variable normal to multiple abnormalities if infection or aneuploidy

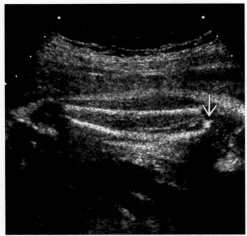

Symmetric IUGR. This patient presented in the third trimester with no prenatal care. By LMP GA 37.5 weeks, by sonographic criteria 33.1 weeks. The proximal tibial ossification center (arrow) is visible confirming that this fetus is at least 35 weeks gestation.

- Echogenic bowel: 16% association with IUGR

MR Findings
- Possible application in evaluation of anomalies
- Useful to confirm destructive intracranial processes in infection
  - Impacts mode of delivery
  - C-section for fetal distress not indicated if brain already damaged

Imaging Recommendations
- Accurate dating essential
  - First trimester: +/- 0.7 weeks
    - Crown-rump length (CRL)
  - Second trimester: +/- 1.5 weeks
    - Biparietal diameter (BPD)
    - Head and abdominal circumference (HC, AC)
    - Femur length (FL)
  - Third trimester: +/- 3 to 4 weeks
    - BPD, HC, AC, FL
    - Distal femoral epiphysis: $\geq$ 32 weeks
    - Proximal tibial epiphysis: $\geq$ 35 weeks
  - Earliest scan is most accurate: Later scans should **never** be used to change dates
- Amniotic fluid assessment
  - **IUGR + polyhydramnios = Ominous combination**
    - High risk for trisomy 18
- Careful search for anomalies: Strong association with aneuploidy
- Look for signs intrauterine infection
  - Ventriculomegaly
  - Hydrops
  - Calcifications
    - Intracranial: Cytomegalovirus (CMV), toxoplasmosis

- Liver: CMV, toxoplasmosis, herpes simplex

Differential Diagnosis

Incorrect Dates
- Menstrual history
  - o Nursing
  - o Birth control
  - o Irregular cycles
- Biometry off by about 4 weeks
- Normal anatomic survey
- Normal interval growth on follow-up exam

Small but Normal
- By definition 10% of pregnancies will be "too small"
- Constitutional: Look at the parents
- Interval growth normal
  - o Fetus remains SGA but exhibits normal growth
  - o SGA with pathology: Interval growth often worsens
- Prior deliveries: Small but well

Pathology

General
- Genetics
  - o Trisomy 18, 13, 10
    - IUGR **not** a dominant feature trisomy 21
  - o Triploidy
- Etiology-Pathogenesis
  - o Syndromes/chromosomes
  - o Intrauterine infection
  - o AIDS embryopathy
    - Vertical transmission
    - Characteristic craniofacial abnormalities: Lateral bossing, hypertelorism, short nose, flat nasal bridge
- Epidemiology
  - o By definition IUGR in 10% of pregnancies
  - o 20% of stillbirths

Clinical Issues

Presentation
- Fundamental problem with fetus
  - o Presents earlier than asymmetric, often early 2nd trimester

Treatment & Prognosis
- If structural abnormalities: Karyotype, infection screen
- Offer termination: Encourage autopsy for specific diagnosis
- If pregnancy progresses with known poor prognosis e.g. trisomy 18
- No monitoring in labor: No intervention for fetal indication
- If pregnancy progresses without clear diagnosis full resuscitation appropriate until cause and prognosis established
- Poor

Selected References
1. Resnick R: Intrauterine growth restriction. Obstet Gynecol 99:490-6, 2002
2. Bromley B et al: Is fetal hyperechoic bowel on second-trimester sonogram an indication for amniocentesis? Obstet Gynecol 83:647-51, 1994
3. Barkin SZ et al: Sever polyhydramnios: incidence of anomalies. AJR 148:155-9, 1987

Asymmetric IUGR

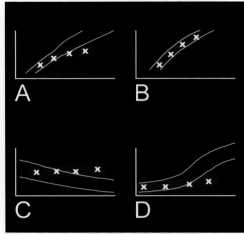

Asymmetric IUGR. Graphic representation of biometry showing EFW < 10th percentile (D) with most marked growth delay in the abdominal circumference (A). HC/AC (C) ratio abnormal as head growth (B) is relatively spared.

Key Facts
- Synonym: Small for gestational age (SGA), intrauterine growth retardation
- Definition
  o Estimated fetal weight (EFW) < 10th percentile **for gestational age**
  o **Asymmetric:** Abdomen < other biometric parameters
- Classic imaging appearance: Size less than expected, low fluid
- Placental insufficiency commonest cause
- **Doppler studies not diagnostic for IUGR but helps guide management**
- Interpretation requires understanding of fetoplacental hemodynamics
  o Abnormal placentation ⇒ increased placental vascular resistance (PVR)
  o Abnormal PVR ⇒ high resistance umbilical artery (UA) waveform
    ▪ Quantified by standard deviation (SD) ratio
    ▪ Peak systolic (PSV)/End diastolic velocity (EDV)
  o Fetal arterial redistribution: "Head-sparing" pattern
    ▪ Flow shunted to cranial contents, peripheral vasoconstriction
    ▪ Decreased renal perfusion ⇒ oligohydramnios
    ▪ Middle cerebral artery (MCA) flow converts high ⇒ low resistance
    ▪ Quantified by SD ratio
  o Increased PVR ⇒ increased RV afterload ⇒ increased RV end diastolic pressure (EDP)
  o RV EDP ⇒ "Kick back" to right atrium
    ▪ Abnormal flow patterns in ductus venosus (DV)
  o Abnormal DV flow ⇒
    ▪ Back pressure to inferior vena cava (IVC) ⇒ reverse flow
  o Umbilical vein (UV) ⇒ pulsatile
    ▪ Intraabdominal first, then in free cord loops

Asymmetric IUGR

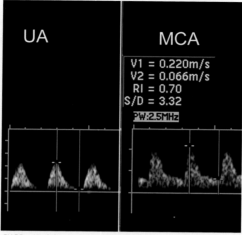

Asymmetric IUGR. Umbilical artery (UA) and middle cerebral artery (MCA) Doppler tracings. UA shows AEDF. MCA Doppler shows conversion to low resistance flow with SD of 3.3. With AEDF the SD ratio cannot be measured. UA SD should always be less than that of MCA.

Imaging Findings
General Features
- Best imaging clue: Fetus with abnormal HC/AC ratio and oligohydramnios
Ultrasound Findings
- Abnormal biometry
- Oligohydramnios
- Doppler changes
Imaging Recommendations
- Monitor amniotic fluid volume: Amniotic fluid index
- Monitor growth: Minimum interval 3 weeks
- **UA Doppler**
  - S/D ratio: "Rule of thumb" SD < 3 in third trimester
  - Absent end diastolic flow (AEDF)
  - Reversed end diastolic flow (REDF)
- **MCA** SD ratio: Should be > UA SD at all gestational ages
- **DV**: Absent or reversed flow with atrial contraction ⇒ poor prognosis
- **UV** Pulsatile flow ⇒ breakdown of fetal circulatory compensation to high placental resistance
- Fetal IVC: Retrograde flow abnormal
- Maternal uterine artery (Ut A)
  - SGA fetuses with normal UA doppler
  - Ut A and MCA abnormal ⇒ 86% risk emergent C-section
    - Ut A abnormal when RI > 0.5 or bilateral notching
    - MCA abnormal when PI < 2.1 SDs from the mean
    - Consider delivery at lung maturity in this group
- **Biophysical Profile** (BPP): Fetal response to hostile environment
- BPP documents acute hypoxia (in increasing order severity)
  - Fetal breathing

- o Fetal movement
- o Fetal tone
- Amniotic fluid: Decrease $\Rightarrow$ chronic hypoxia
- **Nonstress test** (NST): 5th parameter to assess fetal reaction

Differential Diagnosis
Causes Placental Insufficiency
- Primary
- Maternal factors
  - o Hypertension
  - o Collagen vascular disease
  - o Diabetes
  - o Drugs/alcohol/cigarette smoking
  - o Malnutrition

Pathology
General
- Abnormalities in number of placental hormonal factors
  - o Vascular endothelial growth factor, leptin, resistin
- Failure of spiral artery changes in first trimester
  - o Normal low vascular tone in placenta fails to develop
- Reduced placental transfer amino acids/other metabolic substrates
- In severe cases even glucose transport is impaired
- Epidemiology
  - o 10% by definition
    - 3% "normal" pregnancies
    - Up to 25% of pregnancies with past history or maternal factors

Clinical Issues
Presentation
- Late second to early third trimester
Treatment
- Aggressive monitoring
- **2nd trimester management difficult**
  - o Significant risks preterm delivery balanced with
  - o Significant risk intrauterine demise
  - o No single parameter determines decision to deliver
- 3rd trimester with abnormal Doppler, fluid, BPP $\Rightarrow$ deliver
Prognosis
- **Adverse perinatal outcome**
  - o 4 fold increase with IUGR
  - o **Additional** 4-8 fold increase if IUGR + abnormal Doppler
- 50% long-term morbidity especially neurodevelopmental
- "Fetal origins" hypothesis
  - o IUGR babies: Increased hypertension, diabetes, strokes as adults

Selected References
1. Severi FM et al: Uterine and fetal cerebral Doppler predict the outcome of third trimester small for gestational age fetuses with normal umbilical artery Doppler. Ultrasound Obstet Gynecol 19:225-8, 2002
2. Galan HL et al: Intrauterine growth restriction (IUGR): Biometric and Doppler assessment. Prenat Diagn 22:331-7, 2002
3. Hofstaetter C et al: Venous Doppler velocimetry in the surveillance of severely compromised fetuses. Ultrasound Obstet Gynecol 20:233-9, 2002

Macrosomia

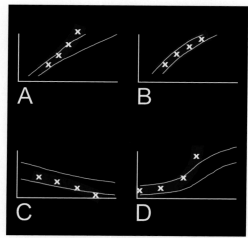

Macrosomia. Growth measurements in patient with gestational diabetes. (A) Abdominal circumference growth reaches > 90th percentile. (B) Head circumference growth remains normal. (C) Low head/trunk ratio reflects large abdomen. (D) Estimated fetal weight is > 90th percentile reflecting risk for macrosomia.

Key Facts
- Definition: **Estimated fetal weight > 90th percentile,** birth weight > 4500 g
- Classic imaging appearance: Fetus is larger than expected, especially fetal trunk
- Often associated with polyhydramnios
- Ultrasound measurements can predict fetuses at risk for macrosomia
- Abdominal circumference measurement correlates best with fetal weight
- **Associated with gestational diabetes**
- Increased morbidity and mortality
- Prenatal prediction leads to earlier delivery and higher cesarean section rates

Imaging Findings
General Features
- Best imaging clue: Large for gestational age fetus with large abdominal circumference (AC) +/- polyhydramnios
Ultrasound Findings
- Fetus seems subjectively large although amniotic fluid is ample
- Abundance of subcutaneous adipose tissue is noted
  - **Truncal obesity** most common
  - Seen best on routine abdominal circumference view
- **Estimated fetal weight (EFW) greater than 90th percentile**
  - Standard charts use multiple biometric measurements
    - Calvarial measurements: Biparietal diameter, head circumference
    - Abdominal circumference
    - Femur length
    - Addition of extra measurements does not improve accuracy
  - **AC usually the first to increase**

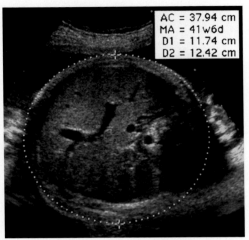

```
AC = 37.94 cm
MA = 41w6d
D1 = 11.74 cm
D2 = 12.42 cm
```

Macrosomia. Abdominal circumference in a 36 week fetus. The AC is measuring 6 weeks greater than expected based on LMP and estimated fetal weight was greater than the 90th percentile.

- o Increased EFW manifested 3rd trimester
- o EFW error rate is higher with macrosomia
    - ▪ 15% vs 10% in normals
- **AC alone may be predictive of macrosomia**
    - o AC < 35 cm
        - ▪ Risk for birth weight (BW) > 4500 g is < 1%
    - o AC > 37 cm
        - ▪ Risk for BW > 4500 g is 37%
- **Idiopathic Polyhydramnios (IP)**
    - o 1/3 of fetuses will be macrosomic
    - o Etiology unclear
    - o Severity of IP does not correspond with severity of macrosomia

Imaging Recommendations
- When AC is greater than expected, follow up for possible macrosomia
- **Growth charts are useful visual tools**

Differential Diagnosis

Beckwith-Wiedemann Syndrome
- Excessive growth starts earlier
- Macrocephaly is more prominent feature
- Anomalies often diagnosed prenatally
    - o Enlarged echogenic kidneys
    - o Macroglossia: tongue protrudes through open mouth
    - o Omphalocele
    - o Polyhydramnios

Other Rare Syndromes Associated With Macrosomia
- Weaver syndrome
- Soto syndrome
- Marshall-Smith syndrome

Macrosomia

Pathology
General
- Etiology-Pathogenesis
  - Polyhydramnios and macrosomia: Suggested etiologies
    - Increased renal vascular flow in larger fetuses
    - Greater fluid flow across larger surface areas (fetus, placenta)

Clinical Issues
Presentation
- Clinical finding: **Fundal height measurement** larger than expected
- Polyhydramnios
- Screening exam for pregnancy at increased risk for fetal macrosomia
  - Gestational and pre-existing diabetes
  - Excessive weight gain during pregnancy
  - Post term pregnancy
  - Prior child with macrosomia
  - Maternal obesity
  - Prior child with shoulder dystocia
  - Maternal birth weight
  - Multiparity
  - Maternal age > 35 yrs

Natural History
- 90% of macrosomic babies (> 4500 g) have no complications

Treatment
- **Early delivery**
  - Associated increased cesarean section rate
    - Elective and in-labor

Prognosis
- Usually excellent
- Complications are related to delivery
  - **Shoulder dystocia (10% of cases)**
  - Asphyxia
  - Hypoglycemia (with gestational diabetes)
  - Low plasma calcium levels (with gestational diabetes)
- Perinatal mortality near 1:100,000 births

Selected References
1. Gilby JR et al: Fetal abdominal circumference measurements of 35 and 38 cm as predictors of macrosomia. A risk factor for shoulder dystocia. J Reprod Med 45:936-8, 2000
2. Sohaey R et al: Idiopathic polyhydramnios: Association with fetal macrosomia. Radiology 190:393-6, 1994
3. Hadlock FP et al: In utero analysis of fetal growth: A sonographic weight standard. Radiology 181:129-33, 1991

Index of Diagnoses

NOTES

NOTES

NOTES

NOTES

NOTES

NOTES

PocketRadiologist®
Obstetrics
Top 100 Diagnoses

Paula J Woodward MD
Chief of Genitourinary Radiology
Armed Forces Institute of Pathology
Washington DC, USA
Adjunct Associate Professor of Radiology
University Hospitals and Clinics
University of Utah
Salt Lake City, Utah
Adjunct Associate Professor of Radiology
University of Maryland
Baltimore, Maryland

Anne Kennedy MD
Associate Professor of Radiology
Director of Women's Imaging
Co-Director of OB Diagnostic Center
University Hospitals and Clinics
University of Utah
Salt Lake City, Utah

Roya Sohaey MD
Associate Professor of Radiology and Obstetrics and Gynecology
Director of Ultrasound
Oregon Health and Science University
Portland, Oregon

With 200 drawings and radiographic images

Drawings: *Lane R Bennion MS*
             Richard Coombs MS
             James A Cooper MD

Image Editing: *Melissa Petersen*
             Danielle Morris
             Ming Q Huang MD
             Cassie Dearth

Medical Text Editing: *Richard H Wiggins III MD*

W. B. SAUNDERS COMPANY
An Elsevier Science Company

AMIRSYS™

AMIRSYS™

A medical reference publishing company

First Edition

First Printing: May 2003

Composition by Amirsys Inc, Salt Lake City, Utah

Printed by K/P Corporation, Salt Lake City, Utah

ISBN: 0-7216-0442-0

Preface

The **PocketRadiologist** series is an innovative, quick reference designed to deliver succinct, up-to-date information to practicing professionals "at the point of service." As close as your pocket, world-renowned authors write each title in the series. These experts have designated the "top 100" diagnoses or interventional procedures in every major body area, bulleted the most essential facts, and offered high-resolution imaging to illustrate each topic. Selected references are included for further review. Full color anatomic-pathologic computer graphics model many of the actual diseases.

Each **PocketRadiologist** title follows an identical format. The same information is in the same place - every time - and takes you quickly from key facts to imaging findings, differential diagnosis, pathology, pathophysiology, and relevant clinical information. The interventional modules give you the essentials and "how-tos" of important procedures, including pre- and post-procedure checklists, common problems and complications.

PocketRadiologist titles are available in both print and hand-held PDA formats. Currently available modules feature Brain, Head and Neck, Orthopaedic (Musculoskeletal) Imaging, Pediatrics, Spine, Chest, Cardiac, Vascular, Abdominal Imaging and Interventional Radiology. 2003 topics that will round out the PocketRadiologist series include Obstetrics, Gynecologic Imaging, Breast, Temporal Bone, Pediatric Neuroradiology and Emergency Imaging.

Anne G Osborn MD
Executive Vice President
Editor-in-Chief, Amirsys Inc

H Ric Harnsberger MD
Chairman and CEO, Amirsys Inc

Notice and Disclaimer

PocketRadiologist®
Obstetrics
Top 100 Diagnoses

The diagnoses in this book are divided into 15 sections in the following order:

First Trimester
CNS
Face/Neck
Chest
Cardiac
Abdominal Wall
GI
GU
Skeletal
Cord
Placenta/Cervix
Twins
Chromosomes
Syndromes
Miscellaneous

Table of Contents

Face/Neck

Chest

Cardiac

Table of Contents

Abdominal Wall

GI

GU

Table of Contents

PocketRadiologist®
Obstetrics
Top 100 Diagnoses

FIRST TRIMESTER

Normal Early Pregnancy

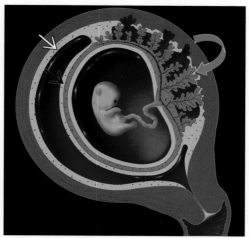

Normal early pregnancy. Diagram depicts the decidual layers which create the DDSS. Decidua parietalis (white arrow) lines the uterine cavity. Decidua capsularis (black arrow) covers the gestational sac. Decidua basalis (curved arrow) fuses with chorionic frondosum to form the placenta.

Key Facts
- Definition: Events occurring in first thirteen weeks of pregnancy
  - Dating based on first day of last menstrual period
- Classic imaging appearance: Intrauterine pregnancy (IUP)
  - **Intradecidual sac sign (IDSS) earliest sign endovaginal (EV)**
  - **Double decidual sac sign (DDSS) earliest transabdominal (TA)**
- Normal early pregnancy milestones: See " Anembryonic Pregnancy"

Imaging Findings
General Features
- Best imaging clue
  - Earliest: IDSS (EV) and DDSS (TA)
  - **Most specific: Yolk sac** (YS) within intrauterine fluid collection confirms IUP
Ultrasound Findings
- **IDSS**
  - Gestational sac (GS) "burrows" into decidualized endometrium
  - **GS eccentric: Within echogenic decidua**
  - **Must follow for development of embryo/YS to confirm IUP**
- **DDSS**
  - Enlarging gestational sac distorts central uterine cavity
  - **Decidua basalis** (DB): Myometrial "base" of sac
    - DB + chorionic frondosum (CF) forms placenta
  - **Decidua capsularis** (DC): Inner, smaller "sac" around embryo
  - **Decidua parietalis** (DP): Outer, decidual lining of uterine cavity
  - DC + DP forms "double" sac
- Yolk sac: ≤ 6 mm diameter
  - **Outside the amnion**
- Membranes

Normal Early Pregnancy

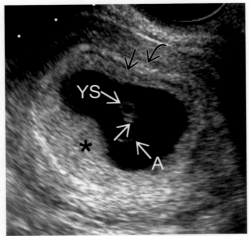

Normal first trimester. EV scan shows "double bleb" sign with the embryo (white arrow) in the amniotic sac (A) immediately adjacent to the yolk sac (YS). An area of thickening (DB + CF) is site of the developing placenta (asterisk). The uterine cavity is a potential space between the DC (black arrow) and DP (curved arrow).

- o Chorion: Thick echogenic
  - ▪ **Gestational sac sonographic term for chorionic sac**
  - ▪ Surrounds amniotic sac, fluid more echogenic
- o Amnion: Thin, inside chorion
  - ▪ Surrounds embryo with anechoic fluid
- • Embryo
  - o Forms **inside amnion**
  - o **"Double bleb" sign**: As early as 4-4.5 weeks
    - ▪ Amniotic sac – embryonic disc - yolk sac
  - o Measurable by 6 weeks
  - o Cardiac activity when ≥ 5 mm
  - o Rhombencephalon
    - ▪ Normal fetal brain structure
    - ▪ Cystic: Precursor to 4th ventricle
    - ▪ Seen as early as 7 weeks
  - o Limb buds
    - ▪ Visible 8-9 weeks
    - ▪ Movement 9-10 weeks

Imaging Recommendations
- • **Standard**
  - o Mean sac diameter: Use up to 8 weeks
    - ▪ Mean of 3 diameters: **Sac only, not chorionic reaction**
  - o Crown-rump length (CRL): Most accurate 6-10 weeks
    - ▪ No biological variation before 10-12 weeks
  - o Record heart rate beats per minute (bpm)
    - ▪ < 6 weeks: 100-115
    - ▪ By 8 weeks: 144-159
    - ▪ > 9 weeks: 137-144
    - ▪ Embryonic bradycardia < 90 bpm

- **Bradycardia < 8 weeks ⇒ 80% loss rate**
- **Additional Options**
  - Nuchal translucency
  - Nasal bones
    - Absence associated with trisomy 21
  - Ductus venosus flow
    - Abnormal waveform associated with aneuploidy
  - Cord diameter (CD)
    - Nomograms created for normal diameter
    - CD > 95th percentile ⇒ predicts embryonic/placental aneuploidy
  - Placental volume: Requires 3D US
    - Placental quotient = placental volume/CRL
    - Statistically significant differences aneuploid to normal

Differential Diagnosis
Pseudosac
- Central in endometrial cavity: **No IDSS**
- Single echogenic rim: **No DDSS**

Pathology
General
- Embryology: Progressive dramatic changes
  - Zygote ⇒ morula ⇒ blastocyst
  - Trilaminar embryo
  - 3D "C shape" embryo: 5-6 weeks
    - Cranial, caudal and lateral folding
  - Closure of neural tube
  - Heart partitioned/aortic arch formed: 8 weeks
  - Development of cord: Seen by 8 weeks
    - Vitelline duct + body stalk + YS + allantois
  - Bowel herniation
    - All bowel returned to abdomen by ≥ 11.2 weeks
    - **Liver never normally out**

Clinical Issues
Presentation
- Missed menstrual period
Treatment
- Prenatal folic acid supplements decrease neural tube defects
Prognosis
- Excellent for live IUP
  - **Demonstration of live embryo 6-10 mm (6.4-7.1 weeks GA)**
    - **0.05% demise**
- Abnormal first trimester: See
  - "Ectopic: Adnexal"/"Ectopic: Unusual"
  - "Anembryonic Pregnancy"

Selected References
1. Metzenbauer M et al: First-trimester placental volume as a marker for chromosomal anomalies: Preliminary results from an unselected population. Ultrasound Obstet Gynecol 19:240-2, 2002
2. Oh JS et al: Gestational sac diameter in very early pregnancy as a predictor of fetal outcome. Ultrasound Obstet Gynecol 20:267-9, 2002
3. Matias A et al: Hemodynamic evaluation of the first trimester fetus with special emphasis on venous return. Hum Reprod Update 6:177-89, 2000

Ectopic (Adnexal)

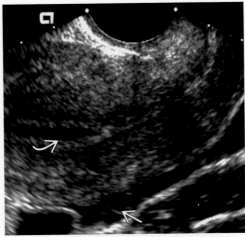

Adnexal ectopic pregnancy. Pseudogestational sac and small complex pelvic fluid in ectopic pregnancy. The endometrial fluid (curved arrow) is in a teardrop configuration. Note there is no double decidual sac sign. A small amount of fluid in the posterior cul-de-sac contains echoes (arrow).

Key Facts
- Synonyms: Tubal pregnancy, ectopic pregnancy (EP)
- Definition: Pregnancy occurring outside of uterus, in fallopian tube
- Classic imaging appearance: **No intrauterine pregnancy (IUP) + adnexal mass + blood in pelvis**
- Transvaginal ultrasound almost always necessary to make diagnosis
- **98% of all EP are tubal**
- Leading cause of maternal death in first trimester: 10% present in shock
- More common in women with history of tubal damage
  - Infertility, prior EP, pelvic inflammatory disease
- Axioms of ectopic pregnancy
  - Best evidence against EP is presence of IUP
  - Absence of IUP significantly increases likelihood of EP
  - Consider EP when intrauterine contents do not look like normal IUP
  - Absence of adnexal findings does not exclude EP but presence of adnexal finding indicates a higher risk for EP

Imaging Findings
General Features
- Best imaging clue: Empty uterus + adnexal gestational sac (not in ovary)
Ultrasound Findings
- Uterine findings vary
  - Empty uterus (thin endometrium)
  - **Decidual reaction** (thick endometrium): With or without cysts
  - **Pseudogestational sac**
    - Teardrop-shaped endometrial fluid that lacks normal double decidual sac appearance (usually blood)
  - Concurrent IUP in cases of rare heterotopic pregnancy
- Adnexal findings vary

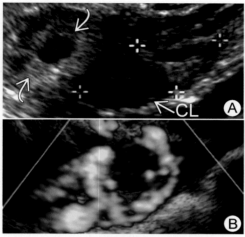

Adnexal ectopic pregnancy. (A) An echogenic ring with faint yolk sac is seen (curved arrows) adjacent but separate from the ovary (calipers). Notice the hypoechoic corpus luteum of the ovary (CL, arrow). (B) Color Doppler shows the typical "ring of fire" seen with ectopic pregnancies.

- o Adnexal mass: Usually heterogeneous, representing hemorrhage
- o Gestational sac: **Echogenic ring**
  - +/- internal anatomy: Yolk sac, living embryo
  - Color Doppler shows "ring of fire"
- o May see no specific adnexal findings
  - Color Doppler may find "ring of fire" when gray scale US is normal
- Ovary findings
  - o Ectopic usually on same side as ovary with corpus luteum (CL)
    - CL may be an echogenic ring, cystic, or solid appearing
  - o **Do not mistake normal corpus luteum for EP**
- Pelvic/peritoneal fluid = blood
  - o Look for **echoes in fluid in posterior cul-de-sac** (high gain settings)
  - o Transabdominal ultrasound (US): Look for fluid in paracolic gutters and Morrison pouch
  - o Complex cul-de-sac fluid may be only finding (85% will have EP)

Imaging Recommendations
- Always perform transabdominal and tranvaginal US
- Correlate US with maternal serum human chorionic gonadotropin (hCG) and progesterone levels

Differential Diagnosis

Normal Early IUP
- IUP not discerned by US because gestational sac too small
- Correlate with hCG level

Endometrial Findings of EP Mimic Early IUP
- Endometrial cysts and pseudogestational sac may mimic early IUP
  - o Look for DDSS and Doppler evidence of single prominent trophoblastic vessel with IUP

Ectopic (Adnexal)

Normal Corpus Luteum of Pregnancy Can Mimic EP
- Corpus luteum in ovary while EP is separate from ovary
  - Use transvaginal probe pressure to show separate areas

Heterotopic Pregnancy
- Definition: Both IUP and EP present
- Rare: 1:10,000 low-risk population, 1:4,000 high-risk population (e.g., fertility drugs)

Pathology
General
- Epidemiology
  - **Increasing incidence** of EP in USA: 5:1,000 in 1970 vs. 2:100 in 1992
  - May be secondary to increasing prevalence of risk factors
  - Increase may be from early detection and treatment of some which may have spontaneously resolved

Clinical Issues
Presentation
- Ultrasound diagnosis may be made prior to symptoms
- First trimester bleeding, unilateral pain, may be severe, 10% in shock
- Physical exam: Palpable adnexal mass in 50%, nonspecific
- **Correlate US with serum hCG levels** (positive predictive value 95%)
  - Normal IUP seen when hCG levels are > 2000 3rd IRP (international reference preparation) (1000 2nd IS [second international standard])
  - If no IUP when hCG > 2000, then ectopic or spontaneous abortion (AB)
  - Opposite does not apply: If hCG levels are low and US findings of ectopic are seen then diagnose EP
  - If hCG is < 2000 and US is negative (no IUP, no EP) then differential diagnosis remains IUP vs. EP vs. AB, must follow serial hCG levels
- Serum progesterone level helps predict normal IUP from EP/AB
  - Less than 5 ng/ml = nonviable pregnancy in 100% (EP or AB)
    - Can do office curettage to determine presence of intrauterine villi
  - > 25 ng/ml excludes EP with 97.5% sensitivity

Treatment
- Laparoscopic surgery +/- salpingectomy: Only choice when ruptured
- **Methotrexate**
  - Stable patients with unruptured ectopic pregnancy
  - EP measures less than 4 cm
  - Multiple doses used and hCG followed (preferred to single dose therapy)

Prognosis
- Good with early treatment
  - 1990s: 9% of maternal deaths from EP (vs. 13% in 1980s)
- 60% of patients will have future IUP
- 6-13% of patients will have future ectopic pregnancy
- Rare progression to trophoblastic disease: Choriocarcinoma

Selected References
1. Frates MC et al: Sonographic evaluation of ectopic pregnancy: An update. AJR 165:251-9, 1995
2. Brown DL et al: Transvaginal sonography for diagnosing ectopic pregnancy: Positivity criteria and performance characteristic. J Ultrasound Med 13:259-66, 1994
3. Nyberg DA et al: Endovaginal sonographic evaluation of ectopic pregnancy: A prospective study. AJR 149:1181-6, 1987

Ectopic (Unusual)

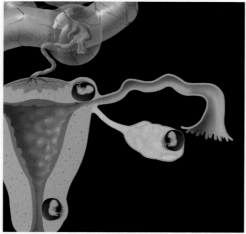

Unusual ectopics. Illustration shows ectopic pregnancies occurring in atypical locations including interstitial portion of tube, cervix, ovary, and abdomen.

Key Facts
- Definition: Ectopic pregnancy occurring in location other than isthmus and ampullary portion of fallopian tube
- Classic imaging appearance: No intrauterine pregnancy (IUP) with a defined gestational sac located in atypical location
- Constitutes **< 5% of ectopic pregnancies**
  - Interstitial (cornual) (2-4%)
  - Cervix (~ 1%)
  - Ovary (~ 1%)
  - Abdominal (rare)
  - Cesarean section scar (rare)
- **Often larger and present later than tubal ectopic**
- At risk for life-threatening hemorrhage

Imaging Findings
General Features
- Best imaging clue: Because of later presentation, a **well-defined gestational sac** can usually be identified
Ultrasound Findings
- No normal intrauterine gestational sac
- **Interstitial (cornual)**
  - Occurs in interstitial portion of fallopian tube
    - Portion which courses through uterine wall
  - Most common location for atypical ectopics
  - Covered by myometrium so grow to larger size than tubal ectopics
  - Located high in fundus
  - Eccentrically located with respect to endometrial cavity
  - **< 5 mm of surrounding myometrium**
  - **Interstitial line sign**
    - Line can be followed from endometrium to ectopic sac
  - Peritrophoblastic flow by color Doppler

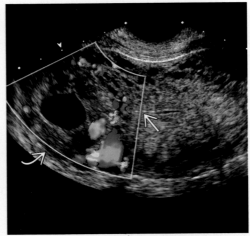

Cornual ectopic. Transverse color Doppler image near the uterine fundus shows a gestational sac located in the right cornua (curved arrow). No normal surrounding myometrium is seen. Note the echogenic line extending from the endometrium toward this sac (interstitial line sign – straight arrow).

- o Treatment usually surgical but medical management has been used
- Cervical
  - o Prior instrumentation risk factor
    - Endometrium is injured adversely affecting implantation
  - o Sac visualized below internal os
  - o Eccentric within endocervical canal
    - Difficult to determine when large
  - o Cervix thins with trophoblastic invasion
    - **Peritrophoblastic flow by color Doppler**
  - o Embryo with heartbeat often present
  - o High risk of serious hemorrhage
    - Cervix predominately fibrous
    - Few muscle fibers for constriction
  - o 80% success with conservative treatment
    - Methotrexate, potassium chloride
  - o Uterine artery embolization, ligation, and/or hysterectomy may be needed
- Ovarian
  - o Rare
  - o **Double ring** or thick, irregular ring
  - o May be exophytic and involve ampullary end of tube
  - o **Echogenic ring in ovary is much more likely to be a corpus luteum cyst**
- Abdominal
  - o Placenta may implant on uterine serosa, mesentery, bowel, or other peritoneal surface
  - o May parasitize multiple vessels
  - o MRI with **MR angiography** helpful for evaluating anatomy and vascular supply

- o May present 2nd or even 3rd trimester
- o Term pregnancies reported
- Cesarean section scar
  - o Implantation within scar
  - o Sac is eccentric to endometrium in anterior wall of lower uterine segment

Imaging Recommendations
- Always document location of sac with respect to endometrium in **both** transverse and longitudinal views

Differential Diagnosis
Tubal Ectopic
- No IUP
- **Extraovarian** adnexal mass
- Uterine pseudosac

Spontaneous Abortion
- May be confused with cervical ectopic
- Sac flattened
  - o Changes shape during exam
- No heartbeat
- No flow with color Doppler
- External os may be open

Normal Early IUP
- Correlate with human chorionic gonadotropin (hCG) level
- Follow-up scan shows normal development

Pathology
General
- Epidemiology
  - o < 5% of ectopic pregnancies

Clinical Issues
Presentation
- Often later than tubal ectopic
- Pelvic/abdominal pain
- Hypotension and shock from rupture

Treatment
- Methotrexate (systemic or injected)
- Potassium chloride injection
- Uterine artery embolization before procedure
- Surgery with potential hysterectomy/oophorectomy if conservative management fails

Prognosis
- Good with appropriate treatment
- Potentially fatal with rupture and uncontrolled hemorrhage

Selected References
1. Sergent F et al: [Ovarian pregnancies: Revaluation of diagnostic criteria]. J Gynecol Obstet Biol Reprod (Paris) 31:741-6, 2002
2. Frates MC et al: Cervical ectopic pregnancy: Results of conservative treatment. Radiology 191:773-5, 1994
3. Ackerman TE et al: Interstitial line: Sonographic finding in interstitial (cornual) ectopic pregnancy. Radiology 189:83-7, 1993

Anembryonic Pregnancy

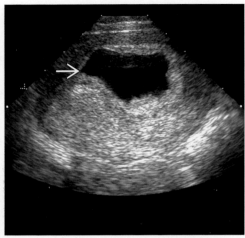

Anembryonic pregnancy. Endovaginal scan shows a gestation sac with mean sac diameter of 30 mm (8 week size). No internal structures are seen, the shape is irregular, as is the decidual reaction (arrow). This is diagnostic for anembryonic pregnancy.

Key Facts
- Synonyms: Blighted ovum, failed early pregnancy, unsuccessful early pregnancy
- Definition: Gestational sac without identifiable embryo when, **by sac size** an embryo would be expected
- Classic imaging appearance: Mean sac diameter (MSD) > 18 mm on endovaginal scan (EV) without visible embryo
- **Normal early pregnancy milestones**
  - MSD 10 mm EV <u>must</u> see yolk sac
    - Some authors use 8 mm as discriminatory sac size
  - MSD 18 mm EV <u>must</u> see embryo
    - Some authors use 16 mm discriminatory sac size
    - Transabdominal discriminatory sac size for embryo 25 mm
  - **"5 alive" rule**: Cardiac activity demonstrable in all embryos $\geq$ 5 mm
  - MSD increases by 1 mm/day
  - MSD at least 5 mm > than CRL

Imaging Findings
<u>General Features</u>
- Best imaging clue: Criteria by EV scan
  - MSD > 10 mm without a yolk sac
  - MSD > 18 mm without an embryo
- **Terminology**
  - Embryonic demise: Gestation sac with nonviable embryo
  - Anembryonic: Failure of embryo to develop or early demise and resorption
  - Consider term "failed intrauterine pregnancy" for both
    - Avoids confusion
    - Simplifies terminology
    - Why blame the ovum with term "blighted ovum"

Anembryonic Pregnancy

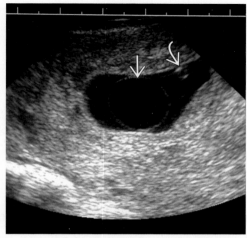

*Anembryonic pregnancy. Endovaginal scan of an intrauterine gestational sac (MSD –
25 mm) shows a yolk sac (curved arrow) and a large amniotic sac (arrow) with no
embryo. This has been termed the "empty amnion".*

Ultrasound Findings
- Irregular sac shape
- Poor decidual reaction
- Sac position low in uterus
- Empty amnion
  - Amniotic sac without an embryo
- Poor color **Doppler** signal around sac
  - Use with caution to support abnormal diagnosis
  - If possibility of normal early gestation, follow up with gray scale rather
    than use Doppler
    - Doppler delivers greater energy with theoretic risks from heating
      and cavitation

Imaging Recommendations
- Confirm absent cardiac activity with two independent observers
- Follow-up if possibility of normal early pregnancy
  - **Know anatomy and developmental stages**
    - Trilaminar structure: "Embryonic disc"
    - "Double bleb": Embryonic disc between amnion and yolk sac
    - Yolk sac and amnion visible > 7 weeks
    - **Embryo inside** amniotic cavity, **yolk sac outside**
    - Yolk sac round in shape, ≤ 6 mm diameter

Differential Diagnosis
Normal Early Intrauterine Pregnancy (IUP)
- Double decidual sac sign (DDSS)
- Thick echogenic decidual reaction
- MSD < 10 mm EV
  - > 10 mm + no yolk sac = failed IUP
- Prominent color flow around sac
- Low resistance high velocity flow on spectral analysis

Anembryonic Pregnancy

- **Remember to use Doppler sparingly in early gestation**

Pseudosac of Ectopic Pregnancy
- **Central** in endometrial cavity
- No DDSS
- Doppler: Absent or low velocity flow
  - Peak systolic velocity < 8 cm/sec

Pathology
General
- General Path Comments
  - 60% spontaneous abortions < 12 weeks due to abnormal chromosomes
    - Trisomies
    - Triploid/tetraploid
    - 45 XO
    - Translocations/mosaics
- Epidemiology
  - **30-60% documented beta HCG elevations end as failed IUP**
    - Pregnancy "diagnosis" biochemical not clinical
  - Early pregnancy failure common with
    - Advanced maternal age
    - History recurrent abortions
    - Poor diabetic control

Pathologic Features
- Chorionic villi present in currettings

Clinical Issues
Presentation
- No fetal heart tones
- Patient perception
  - Diminished breast tenderness
  - Decrease of morning sickness
  - "Doesn't feel like other pregnancies"
- If spontaneous miscarriage imminent
  - Vaginal bleeding
  - Pelvic pain
  - Uterine contractions

Treatment
- "Wait and see"
  - Most will spontaneously abort without treatment
- Suction curettage

Prognosis
- Random event
- No specific recurrence risk
- **Threatened abortion** occurs in 25% first trimester pregnancies
  - Presentation with pain and bleeding after missed LMP

Selected References
1. Sohaey R et al: First trimester ultrasound: The essentials. Semin Ultrasound, CT and MR 17:2-14, 1996
2. Jurkovic D et al: Ultrasound features of normal early pregnancy development. Curr Opin Obstet Gynecol 7(6):493-504, 1995
3. Van Leeuwen I et al: First-trimester ultrasonography findings in women with a history of recurrent pregnancy loss. Am J Obstet Gynecol 168:111-4, 1993

Increased Nuchal Translucency

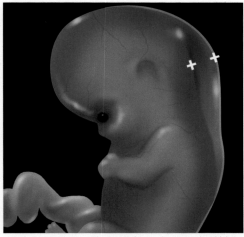

Increased nuchal translucency. The nuchal translucency should be measured as shown above. The calipers are placed such that the largest measurement of subcutaneous fluid is obtained.

Key Facts
- Synonym: Thickened nuchal lucency
- Definition: Increased fluid under skin in back of fetal neck
  - Measured between 11-14 weeks menstrual age
  - Shown to increase fetal risk for **trisomy 21** (T21)
- Classic imaging appearance: **Increased subcutaneous nonseptated fluid** seen on a sagittal image of the fetal neck
- Nuchal translucency measurement can be used as a screening test for trisomy 21 (T21) in certified labs
  - Detection rates of 75-90% reported
- Fetal Medicine Foundation (FMF) has strict criteria for the standard measurement of nuchal translucency (NT)
- Normal range for NT is gestational age (GA) and maternal age (MA) dependent
  - **Measurements > 3 mm generally considered abnormal**
  - < 3 mm may be abnormal depending on GA and MA
- Increased NT places fetus at risk for other chromosome abnormalities, non-chromosomal structural defects, and cardiac defects

Imaging Findings
General Features: Measurement of the NT
- Best Imaging Clue: Appropriately measured NT > 3 mm
- Can be measured successfully by transabdominal ultrasound in 95%
- Crown-rump length (CRL) 45-84 mm
- Good sagittal section of the fetus
- Magnify image
  - Fetus occupies at least 75% of image
  - Incremental increase in calipers of 0.1 mm
    - For example: Can measure 2.1 and 2.2 mm
- **Amniotic membrane can mimic fetal skin**

Increased Nuchal Translucency

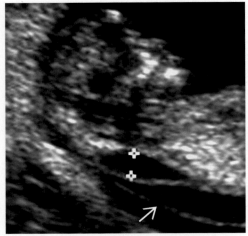

Increased nuchal transluncency in a 13 week fetus with trisomy 21. Note the amnion (arrow) is clearly separate from the measured NT.

- o Wait for fetus to move away from amnion
- Place calipers correctly
- o Maximum NT without skin
- Fetal head in neutral position (not flexed or extended)
- Nuchal cord can mimic increased NT
- NT screening should only be performed by FMF certified labs

Ultrasound Findings
- NT > 3 mm generally considered abnormal
- < 3 mm: Must compare with multiple of median data (NT vs. GA and MA)
- **Risk of adverse outcome increases with increasing NT**
- Septations in the fluid suggests cystic hygroma

Imaging Recommendations
- Look for hydrops fetalis (body edema, ascites, pleural effusion)
- Second trimester anomaly screen with echocardiography in + cases

Differential Diagnosis

Cystic Hygroma
- Neck fluid with septations
- Usually large, can mimic amniotic fluid
- Often with associated hydrops
- 2/3 with chromosome abnormality
- o Turner syndrome (XO) most common
- o Trisomy 21

First Trimester Hydrops Fetalis
- Increased NT + diffuse body wall edema
- Ascites and pleural effusion (not always present in first trimester)
- Prognosis is dismal but some resolve

False Positive From Amnion
- Fetus lying on amnion can mimic increased NT
- Must identify the amnion separate from the fetal skin

Increased Nuchal Translucency

Pathology
General
- Etiology-Pathogenesis (postulated)
  - Abnormal or delayed development of lymphatic system
    - Turner and T21 fetuses have abnormal lymphatic drainage
  - Failure of lymphatic drainage due to impaired fetal movement
    - Musculoskeletal abnormalities
  - Cardiac failure
  - Altered composition of extracellular matrix
  - Fetal anemia
  - Congenital infection
- Associated with non-chromosomal structural anomalies
  - Skeletal dysplasia
  - Cardiac defects
  - Diaphragmatic hernia
  - Omphalocele
  - VACTERL association

Clinical Issues
Presentation
- Incidentally seen during ultrasound performed for another reason
- Seen at chromosome screening examination at a certified lab

Natural History
- May resolve spontaneously
- May progress to second trimester nuchal skin thickening
- May progress to hydrops when severe

Treatment
- Genetic counseling
- Risk of aneuploidy warrants chorionic villus sampling (CVS) or early amniocentesis

Prognosis
- When chromosomes are normal, 90% have normal outcome
- When NT > 99th percentile and normal chromosomes, 8% cardiac defects

Selected References
1. Nicolaides KH et al: Nuchal translucency and chromosome defects, in Diploma in Fetal Medicine Series: The 11-14 week scan. Parthenon Publishing group 1:1-50, 1999
2. Pandya PP et al: Chromosome defects and outcome in 1,015 fetuses with increased nuchal translucency. Ultrasound Obstet Gynecol 5:15-9, 1995
3. Pandya PP et al: Natural history of trisomy 21 fetuses with fetal nuchal translucency. Ultrasound Obstet Gynecol 5:381-3, 1995

Perigestational Hemorrhage

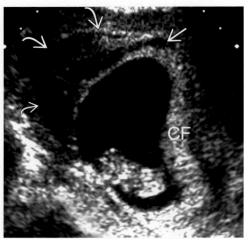

Perigestational hemorrhage. Transabdominal sagittal view through first trimester uterus shows crescent-shaped, hypoechoic hematoma superior to gestational sac (curved arrows). Note the chorionic frondosum (CF) edge has been slightly lifted (arrow). The pregnancy progressed without complication.

Key Facts
- Synonyms: Subchorionic hemorrhage, intrauterine hematoma
- Definition: **Bleeding from chorionic frondosum** (early placenta) in first 13 weeks of gestation
- Classic imaging appearance: Hematoma, of variable size and echogenicity, seen adjacent to gestational sac
- Blood in subchorionic space
  - Between uterine decidua and chorion
- **Small perigestational hemorrhage (PH) has good prognosis**
- Present with **symptoms of threatened abortion**
  - Vaginal bleeding and cramping with closed cervix
  - 25% of all pregnancies with threatened abortion
    - 50% of these pregnancies fail
  - Perigestational hemorrhage seen in 20% of all threatened abortion
- Mechanism similar to marginal abruption seen in 2nd trimester
- Presenting **symptoms may mimic ectopic pregnancy**

Imaging Findings
General Features
- Best imaging clue: Focal hypoechoic fluid collection adjacent to developing placenta and gestational sac in first trimester
Ultrasound Findings
- Appearance of hematoma **varies with age of bleed**
  - Acute hematoma
    - Echogenic or isoechoic to chorionic frondosum
  - Subacute hematoma
    - More hypoechoic and complex
  - Resolving hematoma
    - Liquefies: Sonolucent

Perigestational Hemorrhage

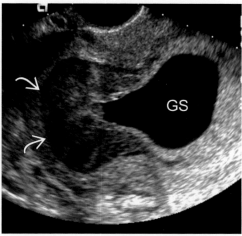

Perigestational hemorrhage. Transvaginal ultrasound of threatened abortion in early pregnancy shows relatively large hypoechoic hematoma (curved arrows) adjacent to misshaped gestational sac (GS) lacking yolk sac and embryo. On follow-up ultrasound, a living embryo never developed, and the pregnancy failed.

- Shape is usually **curvilinear**
  - Extending from edge of early placenta
  - May extend almost completely around gestational sac
  - Blood in subchorionic space
- Large PH **may be mass-like**
  - Significantly compress gestational sac (GS)
  - Mimic anembryonic sac
  - Mimic "pseudo-sac" of ectopic pregnancy
  - **Mimic a second GS**
- **Associated findings are important for determining prognosis**
  - Poor prognosis
    - Absent yolk sac
    - Absent embryo
    - Irregular or low gestational sac
    - Bradycardia $\leq$ 90 beats/minute
    - < 50% attached chorionic frondosum
    - Cervical os dilatation results in miscarriage

Imaging Recommendations
- **Transvaginal ultrasound** for better visualization
- Look carefully at gestational sac features to determine prognosis
- PH may resemble gestational sac or twin

Differential Diagnosis

Chorioamniotic Separation
- Normal separation between amnion and chorion before 14 weeks
- Patient is usually asymptomatic
- Membrane may be seen along fetal surface of placenta
- Placental edges well attached

Perigestational Hemorrhage

<u>Failed, Early Dichorionic Twin Gestation</u>
- Symmetric decidual reaction around second gestational sac
- **May look exactly like small PH**
- Follow-up exam to see if embryo cardiac activity develops in second sac

Pathology
<u>General</u>
- Etiology-Pathogenesis
  o Bleed may originate from chorionic frondosum or decidua
  o Blood can dissect under placenta and around GS
  o May detach GS completely
  o Process often self-limited
- Epidemiology
  o **Threatened abortion in 25% of all pregnancies**
    ▪ 20% with PH

Clinical Issues
<u>Presentation</u>
- Bleeding
- Uterine cramping
- Closed cervical os
<u>Treatment</u>
- If hormone levels normal and ultrasound findings minimal
  o Follow-up scan
  o Patient to be vigilant about seeking care if increased bleeding
- For pregnancy failure (embryonic demise, falling hormone levels)
  o Evacuation of uterus
  o Expectant management and miscarriage
<u>Prognosis</u>
- Guarded when early (no living embryo yet) and PH small/moderate
  o 50% of all threatened abortions abort
- **Excellent when living embryo seen and PH is small/moderate**
  o > 90% successful pregnancy
- Guarded prognosis if PH is large
- Poor prognosis if > 50% of placenta detached or embryonic bradycardia
- **Cervical os dilatation associated with near 100% abortion rate**

Selected References
1. Dickey RP et al: Relationship of first trimester subchorionic bleeding detected by color Doppler ultrasound to subchorionic fluid, clinical bleeding, and pregnancy outcome. Obstet Gynecol 80:415-20, 1992
2. Jarjour L et al: Reliability of transvaginal ultrasound in detecting first trimester pregnancy abnormalities. Fertil Steril 56:202-7, 1991
3. Rempen A: Diagnosis of viability in early pregnancy with vaginal sonography. J Ultrasound Med 9:711-6, 1990

PocketRadiologist®
Obstetrics
Top 100 Diagnoses

CNS

Anencephaly

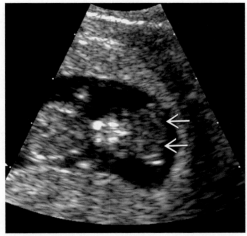

Anencephaly in a first trimester fetus. Coronal sonogram of the head shows a lobulated "Mickey Mouse" appearance of the neural tissue with no cranial vault (arrows).

Key Facts
- Synonym: Exencephaly, **exencephaly/anencephaly sequence**
- Definition: Absence of cranial vault and varying amounts of cerebral hemispheres
- Classic imaging appearance: No cranium or neural tissue above orbits
- Begins as exencephaly (exposed neural tissue)
  - Tissue is eroded by amniotic fluid and fetal movement
- Can be diagnosed in 1st trimester
- Treatment with **folic acid reduces risk of recurrence**

Imaging Findings
<u>General Features</u>
- Best imaging clue: **No calvarium** with flattening of tissues above orbits
<u>Ultrasound Findings</u>
- **First trimester**
  - Neural tissue is still present (exencephaly)
  - Normal head contour is lost
  - Head has an irregular, flattened, splayed appearance
  - Exposed brain has a **lobulated** "Mickey Mouse" or "spiked" appearance
  - Crown-rump length less than expected
- **Second and third trimester**
  - Neural tissue has dissolved
  - "**Frog-like**" appearance when face viewed in coronal plane
  - Polyhydramnios common
    - Secondary to impaired swallowing
  - May have other open neural tube defects (ONTD)
    - Iniencephaly
    - Lumbar myelomeningocele
  - Associated abnormalities

Anencephaly

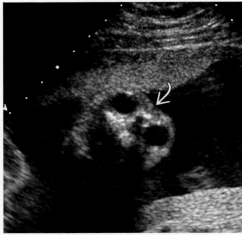

Anencephaly in a second trimester fetus. Coronal view of the fetal face shows two prominent orbits with no neural tissue or calvarium above the orbital ridge (arrow). This appearance has been described as "frog-like."

- Clubbed feet
- Cleft lip/palate
- Omphalocele
- Urinary tract malformations

MR Findings
- Can be used for confirmation

Imaging Recommendations
- Transvaginal scanning in 1st trimester for earlier diagnosis
- **Routine 2nd trimester cranial views detect 100% of cases**

Differential Diagnosis

Acrania
- Defined neural tissue still present
- Brain better seen than normal; secondary to absent skull
- Considered part of anencephaly spectrum
- Lethal

Encephalocele
- Cranium present
- Neural tissue protrudes from defect

Amniotic Band Syndrome
- Defect is asymmetric
- Bands should be visible
- Other body parts often affected

Microcephaly
- Cranium intact

Pathology

General
- General Path Comments
  - Defect is covered by angiomatous stroma (area cerebrovasculosa)

Anencephaly

- Genetics
  - Multifactorial
- Etiology-Pathogenesis
  - Risk factors
    - Folic acid deficiency
    - Methotrexate, valproic acid, carbamazepine, aminopterin (folic acid antagonists)
    - Insulin-dependent diabetes
    - Hyperthermia
  - Embryology
    - Anterior neuropore closes on day 23
    - Failure of closure results in defects including anencephaly, encephaloceles, and iniencephaly
    - Skull complete by 10 weeks
- Epidemiology
  - 1 in 1,000
    - United Kingdom greatest incidence
  - F:M = 4:1

Clinical Issues

Presentation
- Abnormal first trimester scan
  - Can be reliably diagnosed by 10 weeks
- Elevated maternal serum alpha-fetoprotein (MSAFP)
  - **> 2.5 MOM** (multiples of the median) considered abnormal
  - Detects 90% of anencephaly
- Large-for-dates secondary to polyhydramnios

Treatment
- Termination offered
- Preconceptual folic acid should be given for future pregnancies
  - 4 mg/day beginning at least 1 month prior and continuing through first trimester
    - Decreases risk of all ONTD by approximately 70%
  - 0.4 mg/day recommended for **all women** attempting pregnancy

Prognosis
- Lethal
- 2-3% risk of recurrence of any ONTD

Selected References
1. Chatzipapas IK et al: The 'Mickey Mouse' sign and the diagnosis of anencephaly in early pregnancy. Ultrasound Obstet Gynecol 13:196-9, 1999
2. Johnson SP et al: Ultrasound screening for anencephaly at 10-14 weeks of gestation. Ultrasound Obstet Gynecol 9:14-6, 1997
3. Timor-Tritsch IE et al: Exencephaly-anencephaly sequence: Proof by ultrasound imaging and amniotic fluid cytology. J Matern Fetal Med 5:182-5, 1996

Cephalocele

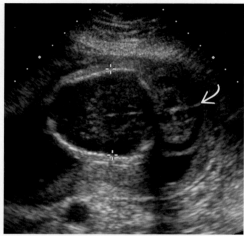

Large occipital encephalocele. Transverse sonogram of the fetal head shows a large posterior cranial defect with herniation of neural tissue (curved arrow).

Key Facts
- Definition: Herniation of intracranial structures through bony skull defect
  - Meninges + brain: Encephalocele
  - Meninges only: Cranial meningocele
- Classic imaging appearance: Cerebral tissue identified protruding through skull defect
- 75% are occipital
- Remainder roughly equal between parietal and frontal
  - Frontal cephaloceles more common in Asian population
- Associated abnormalities in up to 80%
  - Structural, chromosomal, and syndromes

Imaging Findings
General Features
- Best imaging clue: **Skull defect** must be present
Ultrasound Findings
- **Occipital** cephalocele
  - Herniated contents vary from completely cystic to entirely brain tissue
  - **Gyral pattern** can be identified
    - Confirms diagnosis
  - "Cyst within a cyst" suggests prolapsed 4th ventricle
- **Frontal** cephalocele
  - Protruding facial mass
    - Profile view most helpful
  - **Hypertelorism**
  - Herniation may be completely internal into pharynx
    - Difficult to diagnose
- Associated findings
  - CNS
    - Hydrocephalus common
    - Microcephaly in 25%

Cephalocele

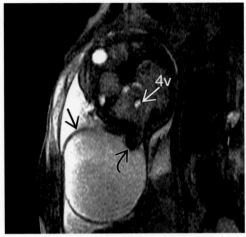

Occipital encephalocele. SSFSE axial image of the posterior fossa shows a large fluid-containing sac (black arrow) with only a small amount of herniated cerebellum (curved arrow). (4V - 4th ventricle, white arrow).

- ▪ Dandy-Walker malformation
- ▪ Agenesis of corpus callosum
- o Body
  - ▪ Facial clefts
  - ▪ Cardiac defects

MR Findings
- Better delineation of anatomy
  - o Involved portions of brain
  - o Coexistent CNS abnormalities
  - o Relationship to vascular structures

Imaging Recommendations
- Follow-up scans to evaluate for developing hydrocephalus
- Monitor head size
- Fetal MRI for difficult cases

Differential Diagnosis
Cystic Hygroma
- Septated cystic neck mass
- Cranium intact
- No neural tissue

Scalp Masses
- Hemangioma, epidermal cyst, cephalohematoma
- Cranium intact
  - o **Must scan from multiple angles** for confirmation
    - ▪ Edge artifact may give erroneous appearance of cranial defect
- May be located anywhere on scalp
  - o Cephaloceles associated with sutures

Amniotic Band Syndrome
- May cause cranial defect and encephalocele
- Bands should be visible

Cephalocele

- Other body parts often affected
  - Large, obliquely oriented facial clefts common association

Acrania
- No cranium

Iniencephaly
- Encephalocele
- Rachischisis involving spine
- Neck in hyperextension ("stargazer" position)

Pathology
General
- Associated with multiple syndromes including
  - Meckel-Gruber
    - Encephalocele, polydactyly, polycystic kidneys
    - Autosomal recessive
  - Walker-Warburg
    - Lissencephaly, hydrocephalus, encephalocele, microphthalmia, cataracts
    - Autosomal recessive
- Chromosomal
  - Trisomy 13, 18
- Genetics
  - Multifactorial
- Etiology-Pathogenesis
  - Embryology
    - Failure of closure of cranial neuropore
- Epidemiology
  - 1-3:10,000 in USA and Europe
    - Majority occipital
  - More common in **Southeast Asia**
    - **Majority frontal**

Clinical Issues
Presentation
- Abnormal first trimester scan
- Elevated maternal serum alpha-fetoprotein

Treatment
- All fetuses should be karyotyped
- Termination offered
- Genetic counseling
- Referral to neurosurgery prior to delivery for surgical planning

Prognosis
- Varies according to severity and associated malformations
- 40% neonatal mortality
- Survivors: 80% neurologic impairment
- Better if skin covered with no neural or vascular tissue
- 2-5% recurrence risk unless associated with syndrome

Selected References
1. Bannister CM et al: Can prognostic indicators be identified in a fetus with an encephalocele? Eur J Pediatr Surg 10 Suppl 1:20-3, 2000
2. Budorick NE et al: Cephalocele detection in utero: Sonographic and clinical features. Ultrasound Obstet Gynecol 5:77-85, 1995
3. Goldstein RB et al: Fetal cephaloceles: Diagnosis with US. Radiology 180:803-8, 1991

Iniencephaly

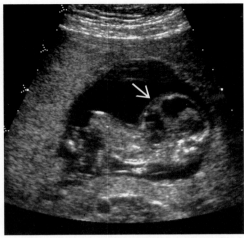

Iniencephaly in a 12 week fetus. There is marked hyperextension of the head (arrow). Also note the body appears small secondary to the shortened neck.

Key Facts
- Definition: Extensive open neural tube defect (ONTD) characterized by triad of
  - Occipital bone defect
  - Cervical dysraphism
  - Fixed hyperextension of head
- Classic imaging appearance: Cervical ONTD with head held in fixed hyperextension
  - "Stargazer" positon
- May be diagnosed in first trimester

Imaging Findings
General Features
- Best imaging clue: Combination of fixed cervical hyperextension, cephalocele, and spina bifida
Ultrasound Findings
- First trimester
  - **Hyperextension** of head
  - Crown-rump length (CRL) less than expected
  - Head appears large
    - Body shortened from absent vertebral bodies
- Cervical spine
  - Fixed exaggerated lordosis
    - > 150°
    - Turns face upward creating **"stargazer"** appearance
  - Large neural tube defect which may extend to involve the thoracic and lumbar spine (**rachischisis**)
  - Short with missing and fused vertebrae
- Other CNS abnormalities often present
  - Anencephaly
  - Microcephaly

Iniencephaly

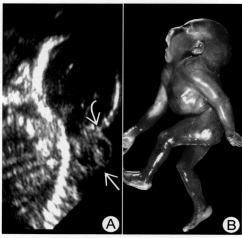

Iniencephaly. (A) Longitudinal image shows hyperextension of the fetal head with discontinuity of the occipital bone (curved arrow) and an encephalocele (arrow). There was an associated rachischisis with the defect extending to the lumbar spine. (B) Photograph shows typical head positioning.

- o Hydrocephalus
- o Dandy-Walker malformation
- o Holoprosencephaly
- Body anomalies
  - o Cleft lip/palate
  - o GI: Omphalocele, diaphragmatic hernia
  - o GU: Hydronephrosis, polycystic kidneys
- Polyhydramnios common

Imaging Recommendations
- Thorough evaluation of spine
- Follow-up examination
  - o Isolated hyperextension without ONTD may resolve

Differential Diagnosis

Cervical Hyperextension
- Head held in extension throughout exam
- **No structural abnormalities**
- Resolves on follow-up exam ⇒ normal outcome
- Persistent finding
  - o 73% normal
  - o 27% unsuspected anomalies at delivery

Klippel-Feil Syndrome
- Cervical vertebral fusion
- Short neck
- Fixed retroflexed position
- **No ONTD**
- Some consider mildest form of iniencephaly

Cervical Meningocele
- Cranium intact

Iniencephaly

<u>Cephalocele</u>
- Cervical spine intact

Pathology
<u>General</u>
- Etiology-Pathogenesis
  - Embryology: 2 proposed theories
    - Failure of anterior neuropore to close (occurs slightly later than in anencephaly)
    - Persistent embryonic cervical lordosis resulting in failure of neural tube closure
- Epidemiology
  - 1-6:10,000 births
  - Higher incidence in United Kingdom
  - F:M = 9:1
<u>Gross Pathologic, Surgical Features</u>
- Defect always involves foramen magnum with 2 types
  - Iniencephaly clausus
    - No associated encephalocele
  - Iniencephaly apertus
    - Encephalocele present
    - Most common type

Clinical Issues
<u>Presentation</u>
- Abnormal first trimester scan
- Elevated maternal serum alpha-fetoprotein
<u>Natural History</u>
- Most stillborn
<u>Treatment</u>
- Termination offered
- Hyperextension may cause dystocia
  - Consider early induction
  - C-section to be avoided
<u>Prognosis</u>
- Lethal malformation

Selected References
1. Sahid S et al: Iniencephaly: Prenatal diagnosis and management. Prenat Diagn 20:202-5, 2000
2. Shipp TD et al: The prognostic significance of hyperextension of the fetal head detected antenatally with ultrasound. Ultrasound Obstet Gynecol 15:391-6, 2000
3. Shoham Z et al: Iniencephaly: Prenatal ultrasonographic diagnosis--a case report. J Perinat Med 16:139-43, 1988

Chiari II Malformation

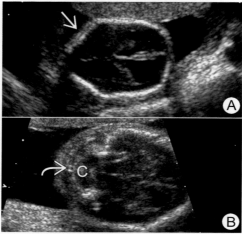

Chiari II malformation. The "lemon" sign describes concave appearance to frontal bones (arrow). There is also ventriculomegaly with a "dangling" choroid. The "banana" sign is the abnormal cerebellar shape (C) with obliteration of the cisterna magna (curved arrow).

Key Facts
- Synonyms: Arnold Chiari II, spina bifida, open neural tube defect (ONTD), spinal dysraphism
- Definition
  - Abnormally small posterior fossa ⇒ symptomatic hindbrain herniation
  - Virtually 100% association with ONTD, usually lumbosacral
- Classic imaging appearance: Obliteration of cisterna magna with curved **cerebellum "wrapped" around brainstem ("banana" sign)**
- Treatment with **folic acid reduces risk of recurrence**
- ONTD often suspected by maternal serum screening

Imaging Findings
General Features
- Best imaging clue: Cranial findings of "banana" and "lemon" signs with ventriculomegaly
Ultrasound Findings
- Cranial findings: > 99% sensitivity for myelomeningocele (MMC)
  - Ventriculomegaly
    - Obstructive secondary to hindbrain herniation
    - ≥ 80% fetuses, may be progressive
  - **"Lemon" sign**: Frontal bones concave
    - Seen in 98% < 24 weeks gestation
    - Always resolved by 34 weeks
  - "Banana" sign: Cerebellum wrapped around brainstem
  - Obliteration of cisterna magna
- Spine findings
  - Splaying of posterior elements on axial view
  - Loss of skin contour axial or sagittal views
  - MMC sac best seen sagittal or coronal sections

Chiari II Malformation

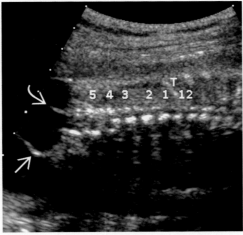

Chiari II malformation. Fetal spine defect. Longitudinal section shows MMC sac (arrow) with contained neural elements (curved arrow). The vertebral bodies are counted from the last rib (T12) to document the level.

- Interpedicular distance increases on coronal section (normally decreases)
  - ≥ 90% MMC (i.e., contain neural tissue), rest are meningocele only
- Associated findings
  - Clubfoot
- **First trimester findings**: New signs described on retrospective review
  - "Acorn" shaped head
    - Dolicocephalic, biparietal diameter (BPD) small
    - "Narrow" frontal bones: Loss of convexity, straight edge
    - Precursor to concavity of "lemon" sign?
    - Sagittal view: Flat occiput
  - Parallel cerebral peduncles on standard BPD image

MR Findings
- Only indicated if considering fetal surgery
- Does not add any information to US diagnosis
- Occasionally of use if maternal habitus limits sonographic evaluation

Imaging Recommendations
- Look for associated **spinal cord tethering**: High resolution linear probe
  - Conus identified as early as 19 weeks
  - Should be at L2-3 or higher
- Look for lower extremity function

Differential Diagnosis

Sacrococcygeal Teratoma (SCGT)
- Usually have mixed cystic/solid architecture
- Spine may be deformed but not open
- Remember SCGT and MMC can occur together

Differential for Hydrocephalus
- Dandy-Walker malformation
- Aqueduct stenosis

- Hemorrhage/infection

Pathology
General
- Genetics: Most sporadic, but increased in trisomies 18, 13, triploidy
- Embryology
  - Failed closure of rostral +/- caudal neuropore
  - Endoderm/mesoderm induction fails
  - No bone/muscle/skin at site of defect
- Etiology-Pathogenesis
  - Risk factors: Valproic acid, aminopterin, maternal diabetes
  - Direct trauma
    - Neural tissue exposure to uterine wall
    - Toxic substances in amniotic fluid
- Epidemiology
  - 1:1,500 live births in USA

Clinical Issues
Presentation
- Elevated maternal serum alpha-fetoprotein (MSAFP)
  - Cutoff 2.5 multiples-of-median: Detects 80%
- Previous affected child
Treatment
- Karyotype
- Offer termination
- Fetal surgery: Selection criteria
  - < 26 weeks gestation
  - Normal karyotype
  - No other anomalies
  - Normal lower extremity function without clubfoot
  - Ventriculomegaly < 17 mm
  - Defect level S1 or higher
- Current research: Management of myelomeningocele study (**MOMS**)
  - Randomized prospective trial to determine efficacy of fetal surgery
- If pregnancy progresses without intervention
  - Prenatal consultation with neurosurgery, spina bifida clinic
  - Mode of delivery controversial
    - C-section may prevent additional neurological impairment
- Preconceptual folic acid should be given for future pregnancies
  - 4 mg/day beginning at least 1 month prior and continuing through first trimester
    - Decreases risk of all ONTD by approximately 70%
  - 0.4 mg/day recommended for **all women** attempting pregnancy
Prognosis
- Depends on level and associated anomalies
- Hydrocephalus, often requiring multiple shunt revisions, significantly impacts long term morbidity

Selected References
1. Buisson O et al: Sonographic diagnosis of spina bifida at 12 weeks: Heading towards indirect signs. Ultrasound Obstet Gynecol 19:290-2, 2002
2. Coleman BG et al: Fetal Therapy: State of the art. J Ultrasound Med 21:1257-88, 2002
3. Jobe AH: Fetal surgery for myelomeningocele. N Engl J Med 347:230-1, 2002

Aqueductal Stenosis

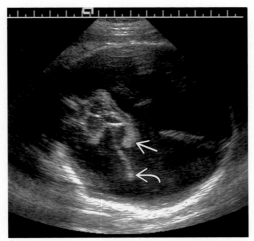

Aqueductal stenosis. Severe hydrocephalus with a dangling choroid (curved arrow) in a fetus with X-linked hydrocephalus. Note the choroid from the other ventricle has fallen through to the dependent side (arrow). The posterior fossa (not shown) was normal.

Key Facts
- Definition: Obstruction at Aqueduct of Sylvius resulting in noncommunicating hydrocephalus
- Classic imaging appearance: Hydrocephalus with normal posterior fossa (PF)
- **Most common** cause of fetal hydrocephalus (~ 40%)
- Multifactorial causation including genetic, infectious, hemorrhagic, neoplastic, and inflammatory
- Associated abnormalities (structural and chromosomal) in 10-30%

Imaging Findings
General Features
- Best imaging clue: **Hydrocephalus with normal posterior fossa**
- **Hydrocephalus**
  - o **Increased intraventricular pressure**
  - o Increased ventricular size **and** increased head size
  - o Noncommunicating: Ventricular obstruction
  - o Communicating: Obstruction of CSF resorption
- **Ventriculomegaly**
  - o **Normal intraventricular pressure**
  - o Increased ventricular size
  - o Head size normal or small
- Anatomy: Aqueduct of Sylvius connects 3rd and 4th ventricles
Ultrasound Findings
- Lateral ventricles measure > 10 mm
  - o Ventricle measured at atrium
  - o Aqueductal stenosis (AS) generally moderate to severe hydrocephalus (> 15 mm)
- "Dangling" choroid
  - o Choroid plexus does not fill lateral ventricle

Aqueductal Stenosis

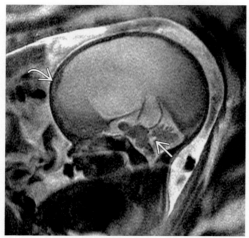

Aqueductal stenosis. Midline sagittal SSFSE image shows severe hydrocephalus. There is a thin mantle of parenchyma seen in the frontal lobe (curved arrow). This was better seen on axial images. The posterior fossa is normal with a normal vermis and 4th ventricle (arrow). Also note large head size.

- o Choroid from opposite side may fall through into dependent ventricle
- 3rd ventricle dilated
  - o Can be difficult to see
- Posterior fossa normal
  - o Cisterna magna can be compressed with severe hydrocephalus

MR Findings
- Better for assessing thinned cortical mantle and any associated CNS malformations

Imaging Recommendations
- Doppler to look for flow in MCA and compressed parenchyma
- MRI to confirm diagnosis
- Follow-up scans every 2-3 weeks for progression

Differential Diagnosis

Holoprosencephaly
- Absent falx
- Fused thalami
- Facial malformations

Hydranencephaly
- No cerebral tissue
  - o Use Doppler
  - o MRI may be necessary for confirmation
- Head size normal

Other Causes of Hydrocephalus
- Chiari II malformation
  - o Abnormal small PF ("banana" cerebellum)
  - o Myelomeningocele
- Dandy-Walker malformation
  - o Cyst in PF

- o Aplasia/hypoplasia of cerebellar vermis
- o Communication with 4th ventricle

Mild Ventriculomegaly (11-15 mm)

- Head size normal or small
- Does not progress
- May be associated with chromosomal abnormality (trisomy 21)

Pathology

General

- Genetics
  - o Sporadic
  - o **X-linked** (Xq28): X-linked hydrocephalus
    - < 5% of AS
    - Males
    - **Adducted thumbs**
    - Mental retardation
- Etiology-Pathogenesis: Incompletely understood
  - o Stenosis may result from inflammation or infection in 50%
    - Disruption of ependymal lining
    - White matter edema
    - Gliosis and fibrosis
  - o Infections: Cytomegalovirus (CMV), toxoplasmosis, rubella
  - o Hemorrhage and tumors also implicated
- Epidemiology
  - o 0.4-1 in 2,000 births
  - o M:F = 2:1

Clinical Issues

Presentation

- May have prior history (X-linked)
- Some not seen until 3rd trimester or neonatal period

Treatment

- Amniocentesis
  - o Karyotype
  - o Infection screen
- C-section only for standard indications
- Ventricular shunting after delivery
  - o Thickness of cortical mantle improves after shunting
- In utero shunting not proven effective

Prognosis

- 10-30% neonatal mortality
- Developmental delay in up to 90%
- X-linked form severe mental retardation
- 4% recurrence risk unless X-linked

Selected References
1. Levitsky DB et al: Fetal aqueductal stenosis diagnosed sonographically: How grave is the prognosis? AJR Am J Roentgenol 164:725-30, 1995
2. Gupta JK et al: Management of apparently isolated fetal ventriculomegaly. Obstet Gynecol Surv 49:716-21, 1994
3. Brocard O et al: Prenatal diagnosis of X-linked hydrocephalus. J Clin Ultrasound 21:211-4, 1993

Dandy-Walker Malformation

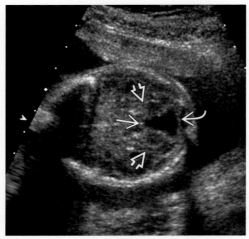

Dandy-Walker malformation. Oblique axial image through the posterior fossa shows a large 4th ventricle (arrow) communicating directly with a midline cyst (curved arrow). The cerebellar vermis is absent and there is splaying of the cerebellar hemispheres (open arrows).

Key Facts
- Synonyms: Dandy-Walker spectrum, Dandy-Walker complex
- Definition: Group of posterior fossa (PF) malformations characterized by
  - Dysgenesis of cerebellar vermis
  - Cystic dilatation of 4th ventricle (4V)
- Classic imaging appearance: PF cyst in direct communication with enlarged 4V
- **Associated malformations common** (50-70%)
  - 50% other CNS
  - 35% body
  - 30% chromosomal
- Care in diagnosing **before 18 weeks**
  - Vermis not complete
  - Normal rhombencephalon in 1st trimester appears cystic
- **Hydrocephalus less common in utero** than postnatal

Imaging Findings
General Features
- Best imaging clue: 4V appears "open" and contiguous with cisterna magna
Ultrasound Findings
- **Classic Dandy-Walker**
  - Agenesis of vermis
  - Hydrocephalus more common
  - PF is large
- **Dandy-Walker variant**
  - Varying degrees of vermian hypoplasia
    - **Inferior** vermian defect
  - Hydrocephalus usually **not** present
  - Diagnosis may be missed

Dandy-Walker Malformation

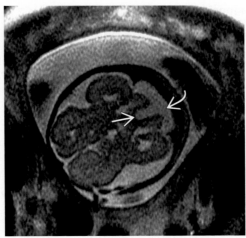

Dandy-Walker malformation. Axial SSFSE image of the brain in a 24-week fetus shows absence of the cerebellar vermis and communication of the 4th ventricle (arrow) with a posterior fossa cyst (curved arrow). The cerebellar hemispheres are splayed apart and small.

- Associated findings
  - CNS
    - **Agenesis of corpus callosum**
    - Encephaloceles
    - Neural tube defects
    - Holoprosencephaly
  - Body
    - Cleft lip/palate
    - Cardiac defects
    - Polycystic kidneys

MR Findings
- Helpful for evaluating vermis and associated findings
- Midline sagittal best view
  - Superior vermis remnant rotated up, over cyst
  - Elevated torcular Herophili

Imaging Recommendations
- Assure appropriate scanning plane
  - **Too steep an angle can simulate** Dandy-Walker malformation **(DWM)**
  - DW variant can be also be under-diagnosed
    - Always scan through **inferior tip** of vermis showing 4V separate from cisterna magna
- Follow-up scan
  - DWM can be over-diagnosed before 18 weeks
  - Hydrocephalus may develop or progress
    - More common after delivery
- MRI for improved anatomic evaluation and associated CNS malformations

Dandy-Walker Malformation

Differential Diagnosis
Mega Cisterna Magna
- Cisterna magna > 10 mm
- Vermis intact
- Thought to be **mildest form of DW spectrum**
- Vast majority considered normal variant, although no long-term studies
- Careful search for other anomalies
Arachnoid Cyst
- Vermis intact
- Displacement of cerebellum with compression of 4th ventricle

Pathology
General
- Associated with multiple syndromes including
  - Joubert
    - DW variant, hydrocephalus, encephalocele, polycystic kidneys, ocular abnormalities
    - Autosomal recessive
  - Walker-Warburg
    - Lissencephaly, hydrocephalus, encephalocele, microphthalmia, cataracts
    - Autosomal recessive
  - Meckel-Gruber
    - Encephalocele, polydactyly, polycystic kidneys
    - Autosomal recessive
- Chromosomal
  - Trisomy 13, 18, 21, Turner syndrome (45XO)
- Etiology-Pathogenesis
  - Environmental factors including maternal diabetes, alcohol, and early in utero infections also implicated but not proven
- Epidemiology
  - 1:30,000 births
  - Higher incidence in utero
  - 10% of infantile hydrocephalus

Clinical Issues
Presentation
- Incidental finding or in workup for hydrocephalus
Treatment
- All fetuses should be karyotyped
- Ventricular and/or cyst shunt after delivery
Prognosis
- 40% mortality in infancy and early childhood
- Intelligence below normal in 70% with classic DW
- Isolated DW variant better but more data needed
- Recurrence risk 1-5% unless associated with syndrome

Selected References
1. Ulm B et al: Dandy-Walker malformation diagnosed before 21 weeks of gestation: Associated malformations and chromosomal abnormalities. Ultrasound Obstet Gynecol 10:167-70, 1997
2. Chang MC et al: Sonographic detection of inferior vermian agenesis in Dandy-Walker malformations: Prognostic implications. Radiology 193:765-70, 1994
3. Laing FC et al: Sonography of the fetal posterior fossa: False appearance of mega-cisterna magna and Dandy-Walker variant. Radiology 192:247-51, 1994

Agenesis of the Corpus Callosum

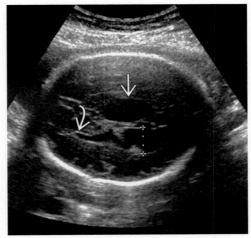

Agenesis of the corpus callosum. Axial image of fetal head shows colpocephaly of lateral ventricle. The medial wall of the ventricle is further from the midline at the frontal horn (curved arrow) than at the atrium (calipers) creating a teardrop shape. There is also an associated interhemispheric arachnoid cyst (arrow).

Key Facts
- Definition: Failure of axons to cross midline and form corpus callosum (CC)
  - May be complete or partial affecting caudal end (body and splenium)
- Classic imaging appearance: Mild ventriculomegaly with **teardrop-shaped ventricles and absent cavum septi pellucidi**
- **50-85% associated defects** including structural, genetic, and chromosomal
  - Most common anomaly seen with other CNS malformations
- Diagnosis easily missed especially before formation is complete (20 weeks)
- In utero MRI very helpful for difficult cases

Imaging Findings
General Features
- Best imaging clue: Teardrop-shaped ventricles most consistent finding
Ultrasound Findings
- **Absent cavum septi pellucidi (CSP) and CC complex on coronal and midline sagittal views**
  - CC forms hypoechoic band on top of CSP
- Colpocephaly
  - Teardrop-shaped ventricles
  - Lateral ventricles widely spaced anteriorly
    - Medial wall of ventricle is further from midline at frontal horn
  - Enlargement of atria and occipital horns
- **Prominent interhemispheric fissure**
- Elevation of 3rd ventricle creating a "trident-shape" in coronal plane
- Gyri in radial "sunray" appearance in sagittal plane
- Doppler shows abnormal course of pericallosal artery
- Associated abnormalities

Agenesis of the Corpus Callosum

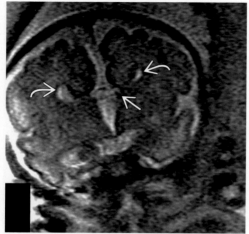

Agenesis of the corpus callosum. Coronal SSFSE image shows complete absence of the CC. The lateral ventricles are widely spaced (curved arrows). There is a "high-riding" 3rd ventricle, which opens dorsally into a widened interhemispheric fissure (arrow).

- o **CNS most common**
  - **Lipomas**: 50% have agenesis of the corpus callosum (ACC)
  - **Arachnoid cysts**
  - **Dandy-Walker malformation** (DWM)
  - Heterotopias and gyral abnormalities: May manifest as asymmetry of cerebral hemispheres
  - Microcephaly
  - Encephalocele and myelomeningocele
- o Body
  - Cardiac defects
  - Genitourinary: Renal and undescended testes
  - Congenital diaphragmatic hernia

MR Findings
- Sagittal
  - o Absent CC
  - o Absent cingulate gyrus
  - o Abnormal radially oriented gyri
- Coronal
  - o Absent CC
  - o Widened interhemispheric fissure
  - o "High-riding" 3rd ventricle
  - o "Trident-shaped" ventricles

Imaging Recommendations
- Meticulous scanning needed to make diagnosis
  - o Often missed or misdiagnosed as hydrocephalus
- If fetus is cephalic, perform endovaginal scan for better evaluation
- **Midline sagittal and coronal** planes often more helpful than routine transverse planes
- Look for associated abnormalities

Agenesis of the Corpus Callosum

- MRI for equivocal cases and detection of other CNS malformations
  - Absence of other abnormalities reassuring

Differential Diagnosis
Mild Ventriculomegaly
- Ventricles will have normal configuration
- Normal gyral pattern
- **CSP present**
Lobar Holoprosencephaly
- Falx may be absent or abnormal
- Fused frontal horns

Pathology
General
- Syndromes
  - Aicardi (DWM, ACC, ocular abnormalities, choroid plexus cysts)
  - Apert, Fryns, Joubert, Meckel-Gruber
- Genetics
  - Most felt to be sporadic
  - Autosomal dominant, recessive, and X-linked described
- Chromosomal (10-20%)
  - Trisomy 18, 13, 8
- Embryology
  - CC forms in midline lamina between 8-20 weeks
  - Develops from anterior to posterior
    - Partial agenesis involves posterior portion (body and splenium)
- Epidemiology
  - 0.3-0.7% of general population
  - 2-3% developmentally delayed

Clinical Issues
Presentation
- Incidental finding
- Discovered in association with other more obvious findings
Treatment
- Karyotype recommended even if isolated
- MRI after delivery
Prognosis
- 85% normal development
- 15% developmental disability
- Poor if associated with other malformations, syndrome, or chromosomal abnormalities

Selected References
1. d'Ercole C et al: Prenatal diagnosis of fetal corpus callosum agenesis by ultrasonography and magnetic resonance imaging. Prenat Diagn 18:247-53, 1998
2. Gupta JK et al: Assessment and management of fetal agenesis of the corpus callosum. Prenat Diagn 15:301-12, 1995
3. Vergani P et al: Prognostic indicators in the prenatal diagnosis of agenesis of corpus callosum. Am J Obstet Gynecol 170:753-8, 1994

Holoprosencephaly

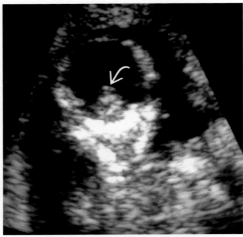

Alobar holoprosencephaly. Endovaginal coronal image of a 12 week fetus shows a large monoventricle. It is surrounding what proved to be fused thalami (arrow) at autopsy (at this age it is difficult to tell fused thalami from brainstem). Of important note, no falx is visualized.

Key Facts
- Synonym: Arrhinencephaly
- Definition: Spectrum of brain and facial abnormalities related to early arrest in brain cleavage and rotation
- Classic imaging appearance: Variable degrees of ventricular fusion with midline facial defect
- Includes both cerebral and facial abnormalities
  - "The face predicts the brain"
- > 50% have chromosomal abnormality
  - **Trisomy 13** (T13) most common
- Dorsal sac may be prominent feature

Imaging Findings
General Features
- Best imaging clue: Single primitive ventricle
- **Alobar**
  - Single horseshoe-shaped ventricle
  - Remaining brain has 3 appearances
    - "Pancake": Flattened at skull base
    - "Cup": Forms partial crescent around monoventricle
    - "Ball": Mantle of tissue encircles monoventricle
- **Semilobar**
  - Some differentiation of occipital horns
- **Lobar**
  - Further differentiation with ventricular communication only between frontal horns
  - Frontal horns appear more squared
  - **Fused fornices**
    - Appears as round structure in 3rd ventricle
    - Best seen in coronal view